CARDIAC REHABILITATION *Explained*

Dr Warrick Bishop
and
Dr Alistair Begg
with
Penelope Edman

SCAN ME

Unlock Your Book Bonuses at
https://drwarrickbishop.com/page/cardiac-rehab-bookbonuses
including Expert & Patient Videos and Worksheets

CARDIAC REHABILITATION *Explained*

an in-depth guide to understanding and navigating life after heart attack, stenting, or surgery

This book is for you, if you

- have suffered a heart attack or other heart event, lived to tell the tale, and want to live as full and healthy a life as possible – or know a family member or a close friend who is in this situation
- want to know more about cardiac rehabilitation and its long-term, life-enhancing benefits
- need encouragement to start or continue a cardiac rehabilitation program
- suffer from any form of cardiovascular disease, and want to live as full and healthy a life as possible – or know a family member or a close friend who is in this situation
- need to know that you are not alone – as a sufferer or a carer or a support person
- want to know what's going on with your heart
- are a doctor, nurse or student looking for a straight-forward refresher or instructive text
- want a book that you can recommend to your patients, family or friends
- enjoy an informative read.

This book is for you if you have a heart.

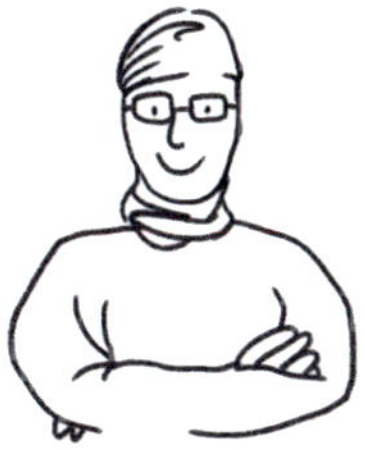

PUBLISHER'S NOTE

The authors and editors of this publication have made every effort to provide information that is accurate and complete as of the date of publication. Readers are advised not to rely on the information provided without consulting their own medical advisers. It is the responsibility of the reader's treating physician or specialist, who relies on experience and knowledge about the patient, to determine the condition of, and the best treatment for, the reader. The information contained in this publication is provided without warranty of any kind. The authors and editors disclaim responsibility for any errors, mis-statements, typographical errors or omissions in this publication.

National Library of Australia Cataloguing-in-Publication entry

Authors:	Dr Warrick Bishop MBBS FRACP Dr Alistair Begg MBBS FRACP FCSANZ DDU
Writer:	Penelope Edman, *PAGE 56*
Title:	Cardiac Rehabilitation Explained
ISBN:	978-0-6452681-4-0 Paperback (Ingram)
ISBN:	978-0-6452681-6-4 Hardcover (Ingram)
ISBN:	978-0-6452681-5-7 Paperback (KDP)
ISBN:	978-0-9756310-0-3 Hardcover (KDP)
ISBN:	978-0-6452681-9-5 Amazon Print (B&W)
ISBN:	978-0-6452681-7-1 (e-Book)
Subject:	Cardiac health care
Publisher:	Dr Warrick Bishop MBBS FRACP
Designer:	Cathy McAuliffe, *Cathy McAuliffe Design*
Illustrator:	Cathy McAuliffe, *Cathy McAuliffe Design*

SCAN ME

For book bonuses visit https://drwarrickbishop.com/page/cardiac-rehab-bookbonuses

dedicated to

those committed to cardiac rehabilitation
who give so generously
so that our patients may recover
as fully as possible
to live as well as possible
for as long as possible

CONTENTS

FOREWORD

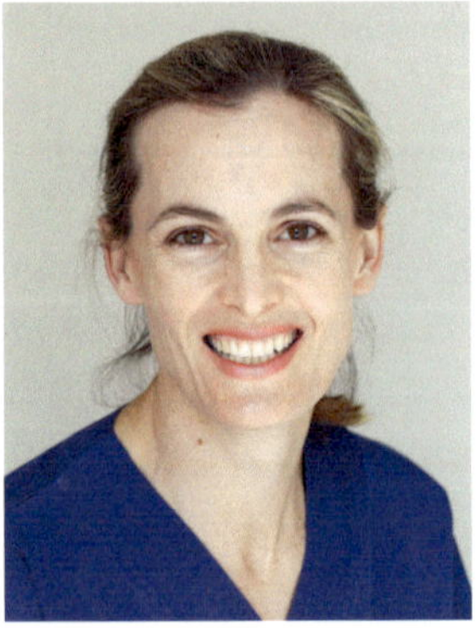

The concept of 'holding someone's heart in your hands' has enthralled many surgeons and physicians for decades, if not centuries.

Restoring blood flow and creating new pathways for blood to travel are amazing medical advances and often profoundly life-altering for patients. These advanced techniques of revascularisation and treatment, however, are merely the first step in a patient's journey back to health and a desirable quality of life. Without a pathway to recover, heal and rebuild, the benefits of surgery and stenting are harder to achieve, difficult to realise and maybe even beyond reach.

Cardiac Rehabilitation Explained is a guide for those patients who entrust us with their lives and, of course, their hearts. When my patients nervously sign the form to consent for major surgery, they want to not only know that the plumbing will be good but also that there is a path back to life, exercise, work, and their families.

Cardiac Rehabilitation Explained is there for these patients.

Many questions are asked prior to the operation, but even more come afterwards as the nerves settle and the 'light switches on at the end of the recovery tunnel'. This book is an excellent reference point for cardiac patients, answering all those questions that are remembered in the middle of the night whilst machines go 'beep' and blood pressure cuffs inflate.

Most of my patients remark, *But doctor, I was perfectly healthy a week ago, and now I have to have my chest cut open for three bypass grafts!* More than half a million Australians have ischaemic heart disease, but the diagnosis is still surprising for some. For these patients, the focus is very much on the upcoming surgery or stenting procedure. Their life is placed on hold to enable them to get through a lifesaving operation. After the initial thrill of *I have survived!*, there is a letdown when they suddenly realise the effort then required to heal and recover. Almost 50 per cent do not return to their normal work capacity after a heart attack, and nearly 25 per cent do not return to work at all. Cardiac rehabilitation looks to support patients back to a healthy lifestyle and the work capacity they desire.

Even in the complex area of cardiac transplantation, cardiac rehabilitation is recognised as critical to patient outcome and quality of life. As the wounds gradually heal, patients realise they have swapped a Morris Minor for a Ferrari. Spurred on by the excitement of a new heart (and high-dose corticosteroids!), the post-operative cardiac transplant patient will benefit from this book, too. For it not only is it about educating the patient on the new medications and a healthy lifestyle, but also the graduated return to exercise, physical activity, and mental preparation for the challenges ahead.

The book takes us on a journey and utilises a wide spectrum of interviews with patients, medical professionals and specialists in rehabilitation sciences. The language is engaging and easy to read, and information is well referenced.

One of my patients once remarked how he read the same newspaper for the first three days after surgery, and each time it was like reading it anew. But as he recovered, his voracious appetite for reading left no book unturned. Combined with the discovery of a fitness tracker, he hasn't looked back unless it is to take a selfie with the other 'mamils' (middle-aged men in lycra) on their Saturday morning bike ride. Now I have the perfect book for him!

EMILY GRANGER MBBS (Hons) FRACS
cardiothoracic and heart and lung transplant surgeon,
St Vincent's Hospital, Sydney, New South Wales

lecturer
Clinical Medical School at St Vincent's Hospital,
the University of Notre Dame

member
Royal Australasian College of Surgeons

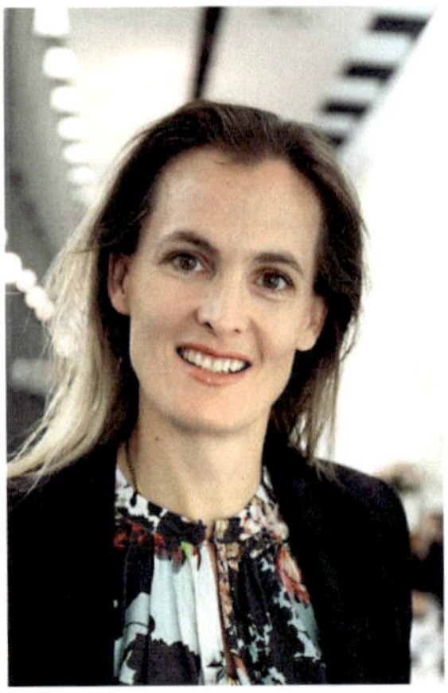

Dr Emily Granger has performed more than 3000 general cardiothoracic operations and more than 300 heart and lung transplants.

Emily completed her medical degree at the University of Queensland and her surgical fellowship with the Royal Australasian College of Surgeons (RACS) in 2006. She is involved with the NSW Organ Tissue Donation Service and Deceased Donor Organ Procurement and, in 2014, was involved in the world's first successful 'donation after circulatory death' heart transplant. Since then, the Transplant Unit at St Vincent's Hospital has performed 80 procedures of this type.

Dr Granger lectures at the Clinical Medical School at St Vincent's Hospital and the University of Notre Dame, and is active in teaching medical students, junior doctors, and trainee surgeons. She is an instructor with the RACS and involved with the RACS NSW State Regional Committee. In 2017, she was appointed to the Board of Cardiothoracic Surgical Examiners. She is president of the Australian and New Zealand Society of Cardiac and Thoracic Surgeons (ANZSCTS).

REFERENCES

Cardiac Rehabilitation Explained has been informed by

National Heart Foundation of Australia and Cardiac Society of Australia and New Zealand: Guidelines for the Prevention, Detection, and Management of Heart Failure in Australia 2018

NHFA CSANZ Heart Failure Guidelines Working Group John J. Atherton, Andrew Sindone, Carmine G. De Pasquale, Andrea Driscoll, Peter S. MacDonald, Ingrid Hopper, Peter M. Kistler, and others.

Heart, Lung and Circulation, Vol. 27, Issue 10, p1123–1208
Published in issue: October 2018
© 2018 National Heart Foundation of Australia. Published by Elsevier B.V. on behalf of the Australian and New Zealand Society of Cardiac and Thoracic Surgeons (ANZSCTS) and the Cardiac Society of Australia and New Zealand (CSANZ).

A Pathway to Cardiac Recovery
Standardised program content for Phase II Cardiac Rehabilitation

Working group: Institute for Physical Activity, Deakin University, Dr Susie Cartledge, Dr Emma Thomas, Professor Ralph Maddison; Heart Foundation and Nutrition, Deakin University, Kerry Hollier, Roni Beauchamp, Dr Sue Forrest, Eugene Lugg, Expert Advisory Group (EAG), Professor Robyn Gallagher, Dr Adrienne O'Neil, Cate Ferry, Professor Nicholas Cox, Professor Lis Neubeck, Professor Robyn Clark, Stephen Woodruffe, Emma Boston, Kim Gray, A/Professor Julie Redfern, Beth Meertens, Dr Bridget Abell, Dr Carolyn Astley, Maria Sheehan, A/Professor Rosemary Higgins, Content experts (outside of EAG), Cia Connell (Heart Foundation), Sian Armstrong (Heart Foundation), Sarah White (QUIT Victoria).

© 2019 National Heart Foundation of Australia
https://www.heartfoundation.org.au/getmedia/006fd247-6163-4d04-9b85 9e90a5adbea0/A_Pathway_to_Phase_II_Cardiac_Recovery_(Full_Resource)-(3).pdf

and the paper about how the resource was written:
Development of standardised programme content for phase II cardiac rehabilitation programmes in Australia using a modified Delphi process

Susie Cartledge, Emma Thomas, Kerry Hollier, R Maddison
BMJ Journals (Open) volume 9, issue 12 https://bmjopen.bmj.com/content/9/12/e032279

Improving the Monitoring of Cardiac Rehabilitation Delivery and Quality: A Call to Action for Australia

Emma Thomas, MPH, Carolyn Astley, PhD, Robyn Gallagher, PhD, Rachelle Foreman, MPhil, Julie Anne Mitchell, MPH, Sherry L. Grace, PhD, Dominique A. Cadilhac, PhD, Stephen Bunker, PhD, Alexander Clark, MPH, Adrienne O'Neil, PhD.

Received 25 May 2019; online published-ahead-of-print 16 August 2019
(editorial) *Heart, Lung and Circulation* (2020) 29, 1–4
https://doi.org/10.1016/j.hlc.2019.07.013
© 2019 Australian and New Zealand Society of Cardiac and Thoracic Surgeons (ANZSCTS) and the Cardiac Society of Australia and New Zealand (CSANZ). Published by Elsevier B.V. All rights reserved.

The BACPR (British Association for Cardiovascular Prevention and Rehabilitation) Standards and Core Components for Cardiovascular Disease Prevention and Rehabilitation 2017

https://www.bacpr.com/resources/BACPR_Standards_and_Core_Components_2017.pdf

Cochrane Library

Cochrane Reviews – cardiac rehabilitation
https://www.cochranelibrary.com

Australian Cardiovascular Health and Rehabilitation Association (ACRA) Core Components of Cardiovascular Disease Secondary Prevention and Cardiac Rehabilitation 2014

Stephen Woodruffe, Lis Neubeck, PhD, Robyn A. Clark, PhD, Kim Gray, Cate Ferry, Jenny Finan, MN, Sue Sanderson, Tom G. Briffa, PhD.

Online published-ahead-of-print 12 January 2015
(review) *Heart, Lung and Circulation* (2015) 24, 430–441 1443-9506/04/
http://dx.doi.org/10.1016/j.hlc.2014.12.008
© 2015 Australian and New Zealand Society of Cardiac and Thoracic Surgeons (ANZSCTS) and the Cardiac Society of Australia and New Zealand (CSANZ). Published by Elsevier Inc. All rights reserved.

Recommendations for participation in competitive and leisure time sport in athletes with cardiomyopathies, myocarditis, and pericarditis: position statement of the Sport Cardiology Section of the European Association of Preventive Cardiology (EAPC)

Antonio Pelliccia, Erik Ekker Solberg, Michael Papadakis, Paolo Emilio Adami, Alessandro Biffi, Stefano Caselli, Andrè La Gerche, Josef Niebauer, Axel Pressler, Christian M. Schmied10, Luis Serratosa, Martin Halle, Frank Van Buuren, Mats Borjesson, Francois Carrè, Nicole M. Panhuyzen-Goedkoop, Hein Heidbuchel, Iacopo Olivotto, Domenico Corrado, Gianfranco Sinagra, and Sanjay Sharma.

Received 5 August 2017; revised 8 March 2018; editorial decision 19 October 2018; accepted 20 October 2018; online publish-ahead-of-print 14 December 2018
European Society of Cardiology, European Heart Journal (2019) 40, 19-23. (doi:10.1093/eurheartj/ehy730) Special article, Sports cardiology

Cardiac rehabilitation: a comprehensive review

Scott A Lear and Andrew Ignaszewski

Published online: 10 September 2001. Curr Control Trials Cardiovasc Med 2001, 2:221-232 © 2001 BioMed Central Ltd (Print ISSN 1468-6708; Online 1468-6694)

Austroads and the National Transport Commission, Assessing Fitness to Drive

https://austroads.com.au/

Qantas Group Medical Travel Clearance Guidelines

https://www.qantas.com.au/infodetail/flying/beforeYouTravel/mediform.pdf

other websites:

American Heart Association	https://www.heart.org
Australian Institute of Health and Welfare	https://www.aihw.gov.au
Harvard Publishing, Harvard Medical School	https://www.health.harvard.edu
Healthy Heart Network	https://healthyheartnetwork.com
Heart Foundation (Australia)	https://www.heartfoundation.org
Heart of the Nation	https://heartofthenation.com.au
Heart Research Institute	https://www.hri.org.au
National Heart, Lung and Blood Institute	https://www.nhlbi.nih.gov
National Library of Medicine (National Centre for Biotechnology Information)	https://www.ncbi.nlm.nih.gov
Nutrition for Life Healthcare	https://nutritionforlifehealthcare.com.au
ResearchGate	https://www.researchgate.net
The Lancet	https://www.thelancet.com
The New England Journal of Medicine	https://www.nejm.org
Victor Chang Cardiac Research Institute	https://www.victorchang.edu.au
World Economic Forum	https://www.weforum.org
World Health Organization	https://www.who.int
World Heart Federation	https://world-heart-federation.org

books, text:

Begg, Alistair; *What's Wrong With My Heart?* (unpublished text)

Bishop, Warrick; *Have You Planned Your Heart Attack?* (2016)

Bishop, Warrick; *Atrial Fibrillation Explained* (2019)

Bishop, Warrick; *Cardiac Failure Explained* (2020)

It does not matter how slowly you go as long as you do not stop.

Confucius

introduction

In 2018, Ron, aged 66, was living what seemed a healthy enough life. At 180 cm tall, he weighed around 78 kg. He didn't smoke, wasn't diabetic, ate mostly vegetarian, drank a bottle of wine over two days on the weekend and consumed no alcohol on the remaining five days. He rarely ate junk food and consistently observed the 5/2 fast diet, having done so for three years. At least three days a week, he walked for an hour or more.

On a Monday morning in August 2018, he had a heart attack.

PATIENT'S PERSPECTIVE ♥

a journey for which I was not prepared

Rehabilitation after heart surgery was not a journey for which I was prepared. My surgery was necessitated by an unforeseen heart attack, and it was only then that I discovered I had serious heart disease. There was little time to learn what the surgery would involve (four coronary artery bypass grafts). There was no time to ask about or consider what it would be like post-surgery.

When I woke from surgery and discovered the state my body was in, I really confronted what lay ahead and retrospectively learned what had led to this. For a person who regularly walked an hour a day, ate a well-balanced diet and considered himself fit and healthy, I was reduced to an exhausted shell of my former self.

In the immediate aftermath of surgery, my rehabilitation was a medical one and began in intensive care. When I regained consciousness, a breathing tube was removed from my throat and replaced with prongs fixed in my nose to support my oxygen intake. A tube remained inserted into a vein in my neck and a catheter to drain my bladder was connected. There was a tube inserted in my wrist, two drains inserted through my lower chest wall to drain excess fluid and a canula fixed in my arm on the inside of my elbow.

I was attached to a drip supported on a wheeled metal frame beside my bed. For a number of days this drip and metal frame were my annoying companions whenever I ventured from my bed. Electrical nodes were plastered all over my chest, attached by wires to a portable monitoring device that also went with me whenever I left my bed. This device was particularly difficult to keep dry when, after a couple of days of recovery, and to my great relief, I was allowed to shower. Frequently, I was fitted with a face mask nebuliser to help improve the condition of my lungs and my breathing. I didn't understand at first why my lungs were an issue until I was told that during surgery my heart and lungs were effectively shut down and I was maintained on a heart lung device.

For the first day or so I had a self-operated handset to give myself controlled doses of pain relief. Other medications by both tablet and injection were delivered to me throughout the day and night and my blood pressure was taken every few hours. Though understandable for safety reasons, I became tired of confirming my name and date of birth at every nursing visit. Being unable to use my arms or upper body to roll over in bed contributed to my inability to get much sleep. I also discovered that frequent interruptions meant that sound sleep was not key to my hospital rehabilitation.

Within a few days, I was visited by a cardiac rehabilitation nurse and encouraged to get out of bed, spend time sitting in a chair, and as soon as possible begin walking around the ward. I was also shown a series of breathing exercises and told to repeat them a number of times each hour. This involved a series of deep breaths followed by a couple of 'huffs' to expel the air in my lungs through my open mouth. Then came the painful part which was to cough strongly from my lungs. Despite supporting my breastbone (sternum) by clutching a folded towel to my chest, this brought pain and an anticipatory fear of damaging my chest wound where the bone had not had time to heal.

Because of the amount of time spent in bed or sitting uncomfortably in the bedside chair and the consequent risk of deep vein thrombosis, I had to wear pressure socks for weeks after my surgery. These socks were almost impossible to put on and take off without assistance, given the constraints on using my upper body and arms because of my still-healing breastbone. There were also ankle rotations, knee lifting and buttock squeezing exercises to do (if I remembered to do them). I might even inadvertently have ended up strengthening my pelvic floor muscles, though constipation remained a problem!

Prior to discharge from hospital, my recovery status was assessed by a cardiac rehabilitation nurse. This involved an interview, the usual tests (such as blood pressure) and a walking assessment up and down a marked-out section of the ward corridor.

When I was discharged, I was meant to continue some of the hospital exercises at home, along with an additional program of exercises. I had never been one for exercise routines and I felt totally exhausted from the impacts of major surgery. It took considerable will power and my partner's hectoring to comply to a reasonable level with the program.

Fortunately, frequent walking was highly recommended as the best initial rehabilitation exercise after heart surgery, and I had always been a walker. The advice was to keep to flat or gentle grade routes, and with my initially diminished lung function I found this necessary. Before my heart surgery, I had never experienced any diminishment of my lung function and could walk up quite steep hills without puffing. I became quite concerned and stressed at having to catch my breath with anything more than the gentlest of exercise and feared that this was to be my new normal. I gained an inkling of what it might be like to have emphysema. Fortunately, over a couple of months my lung function returned more or less to normal. My appetite, normally healthy, was diminished for a few weeks and I slept a lot.

The hospital provided me with a cardiac rehab booklet with guidelines on returning progressively to everyday activity, covering each week for the first 12 weeks after discharge. Some of the examples given were specific for certain occupations or recreational activities that a person might be returning to, for example farming, golfing, fishing, woodworking, as well as household tasks such as making the bed, ironing, and vacuuming. It was reassuring to be advised that by week four I could begin to practice my putting, develop photos, hang light washing on the line and resume gentle sexual activity with a familiar partner provided I did not "assume the upper dominant position"! Apparently, an unfamiliar partner might induce anxiety. By week eight I could be dancing rock and roll or square dancing. More usefully, and with the approval of my cardiovascular surgeon at my six-week post discharge clinic, I was given the all clear to drive and travel.

Three weeks after discharge from hospital, I commenced a six-week program of rehabilitation organised and run by cardiac rehabilitation nurses. The program was run at a facility on Hobart's eastern shore set up for rehabilitation purposes. Each 2.5-hour session was divided into two parts. The session started with registration and an introduction and explanation of the circuit of exercises new participants would undertake.

Some participants were already part way through their six-week program. Observing their familiarity with the exercise circuit helped me catch on to what was expected. Participants were also in various states of health and physical capacity, so we each received personal attention on what level of exercise we should do and on how to pace ourselves safely as our physical recovery progressed.

Most exercises in the circuit were set for a one-minute duration before moving to the next exercise. Exercises included simple pacing up and down, stepping up and down on a set of steps, raising each knee in turn to waist height, using dumbbells and a light-weight bar weight.

The final part of the program involved using an exercise bike or walking machine. The length of time spent on these was adjusted depending on the individual circumstances of each of the participants. My initial fear was that this seemed much too strenuous after recent heart surgery, and that my heart would not cope. Both machines allowed for an adjustment of the difficulty in using them and tracked my heart rate through the hand grips. I was very concerned to see my heart rate get up to over 140 bpm, imagining at any minute my heart would explode in some catastrophic fashion. The staff monitored how strenuously I participated in each exercise and reassured me that the level of exercise was not only safe but beneficial. Each week of the program I gained in strength and confidence.

Once the exercise session was completed, we reconvened in a meeting room for an information and discussion session. Two nurses shared the role of running these sessions, which each week focussed on a different aspect of heart disease, healthy living, and dealing with recovery from the physical and psychological impacts of heart surgery. Probably each of us found some aspects more relevant than others but, overall, I found the information interesting.

I learned a lot more about how my heart functioned and what had been involved in my bypass surgery. Diet and exercise were also covered as was the emotional impacts of treatment for heart disease. This part of the program was a little stilted, perhaps because of the preponderance of men, poor communicators of feelings at the best of times. No-one seemed to have much to volunteer on how they were coping emotionally, even though statistically we were told something like 30 per cent of heart surgery patients were vulnerable to post-operative depression.

I expressed my fear of going on remote bushwalking and camping trips in case my surgery failed. Another participant suggested that since I wouldn't be nervous to use my car after it came back from the mechanic, I should therefore trust the surgeon's expertise in fixing my heart. Really, though, it was my faith in my heart rather than in the surgeon that was challenged.

Participants who had had heart surgery were jokingly referred to as the "zippers", referring to the scar down the centre of our chests. However, not all participants were bypass surgery patients. A number of people had received stents and one person had received a valve replacement. Their different procedures and recovery paths were interesting. Who knew that pig valves specially developed in Mexico could end up in human hearts?

Most of the information in the sessions was pertinent to everyone, with some relevant to individual circumstances. All but one of the participants were men and to my surprise – perhaps betraying a stereotype I had assumed – only a few participants tended to be obese. There were, however, quite a few smokers.

Because each participant began the program a few weeks after their particular hospital discharge, each week there were people commencing the program and people completing it. For this reason, although there was a friendly atmosphere, particularly encouraged by the enthusiasm and friendliness of the nurses, participants mostly kept to themselves.

The cardio rehab program was well run and developed my confidence in how far I could exert myself. It provided useful information on the procedures we participants had been through, healthy eating, exercise and other related information. I was surprised only a few of the participants matched the stereotype of obese, diabetic smokers. But neither did I. My last session was held on 17 October. While the on-going journey has not been smooth, I am grateful for the support and encouragement and learning received during the rehabilitation. I continue living as healthily as I can.

towards a healthier life

Regular and ongoing contact with a patient's cardiologist and GP ensures that everything possible is done to restore function after a cardiac event or diagnosis. Any lessening of ongoing symptoms in daily life improves quality of life and reduces the risk of another event. Such activities, education and support – whether these are through programs at a hospital or medical centre, or at home – mean a healthier life for the patient and a happier life for those close to the patient.

This is the essence of cardiac rehabilitation, and this is what we explore in *Cardiac Rehabilitation Explained.*

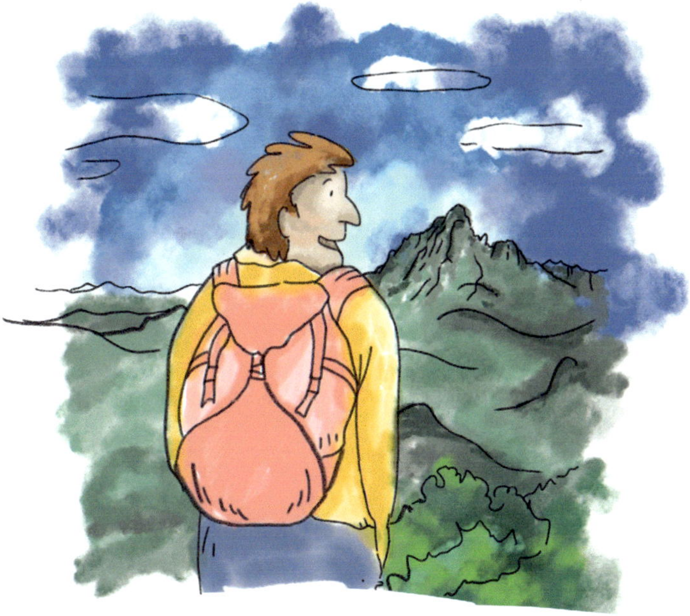

"I expressed my fear of going on remote, bushwalking, and camping trips in case my surgery failed ... Really, it was my faith in my heart, rather than the surgeon that was challenged."

Survivors of a cardiac event need specialised treatment and help to prevent further problems.

chapter 1

A SURVIVAL GUIDE

A cardiac event is not a planned occurrence in a person's life. It comes 'out of the blue', like a car accident or some other form of unexpected trauma. People who survive a cardiac event need specialised treatment and professionals around them who understand what they've been through and what the new journey of life might hold.

A significant part of this unexpected turn is looking to the future to try to prevent more problems, future-proofing the person from another heart attack, further surgery, cardiac failure, or other heart problem – in other words, from cardiovascular disease (CVD).

The term, cardiovascular disease, covers several conditions associated with the heart and blood vessels and most commonly includes coronary artery disease, heart failure and stroke.

Even in this era of COVID pandemic, CVD is the most common cause of death in the world[1] and remains one of the most common causes of hospitalisations in the western world[2]. Globally, it claims an estimated 17.79 million lives a year, about 31 per cent of all deaths[3].

The World Health Organisation says that four out of five CVD deaths are due to heart attacks and strokes, and one-third of these deaths occur prematurely in people under 70 years of age[4].

Using Australian statistics,

- one Australian dies of CVD every 12 minutes
- about 50,000 Australians die of heart disease each year[5]
- CVD affects about one in six Australians and two out of three families.

Most people would have a friend or a relative who has cardiovascular disease. Many of the premature deaths are preventable.

The purpose of cardiac rehabilitation (CR or rehab) is to **equip and encourage people to live life to the fullest again after a cardiac diagnosis, or after the person has suffered a cardiac event or undergone a procedure**.

Key to this is what is called 'secondary prevention of cardiovascular disease', the prevention of a 'second' event, especially of heart attack and stroke, through drug therapy, education, and counselling[6].

Evidence of benefits from rehab is robust and has been demonstrated reliably around the world. As well as helping keep a coronary heart disease patient alive longer, rehab

- reduces the number of hospital re-admissions[7] the person might experience,
- improves the person's functional capacity, which impacts
  - the person's quality of life and
  - financial considerations such as return to work.

cardiac rehabilitation

So, what is this cardiac rehabilitation?

The World Health Organization defines cardiac rehabilitation as

> *"the coordinated sum of activities required to influence favorably the underlying cause of cardiovascular disease, as well as to provide the best possible physical, mental and social conditions, so that the patients may, by their own efforts, preserve or resume optimal functioning in their community and through improved health behavior, slow or reverse progression of disease."*[8]

What this means in practice is that cardiac rehabilitation is a journey to improve the person's health through organised, coordinated hospital or centre-based programs, and/or a schedule of activities undertaken at home. Regardless of where and how these activities are conducted, they are designed to assist with the healing process and the person's ongoing engagement with life. Participation not only improves physical health and quality of life but also equips and supports the person to develop the necessary skills to successfully self-manage. Ideally, rehab is tailored to the individual – incorporating the person's health, physical and mental capabilities, cultural needs, and other personal preferences.

Anyone who has suffered a cardiac event or received a diagnosis knows how frightening and confusing the experience is. Often, it occurs suddenly. The person is overwhelmed with instructions and new medicines. And there are so many questions. The world has suddenly changed, and the future becomes very uncertain. Help is needed.

survival game plan

Australian cardiac rehabilitation specialist Dr Alistair Begg says that rehab is incredibly important not only for the patient but those closely associated with the person.

> *"Cardiac rehabilitation is the whole process that picks up the pieces after a cardiac event. Someone has had a heart attack or comes into the hospital for an operation, and that person has received the initial treatment.* ***Cardiac rehabilitation involves the full support and education and the physical, mental and social conditioning that occurs after that event.*** *Cardiac rehabilitation takes the patient through the whole journey after the initial visit to the hospital or the cardiac event.* ***It is a complex and multi-faceted journey.****"*[9]

Dr Begg said that cardiologists were ideally placed to help 'pick up the pieces'.

> *"Not only do cardiologists deliver the acute treatment, but they can also supervise the longer-term recovery process. Using our knowledge, we are able to*
>
> - *educate patients*
> - *reassure them*
> - *guide them into the areas they need to work on, and*

- *coordinate the involvement of the range of allied health professionals required, such as*
  > *nurses*
  > *dietitians*
  > *nutritionists*
  > *exercise professionals, and*
  > *mental health practitioners."*

He said that in picking up the pieces for a shell-shocked patient, the cardiologist needed to look at **why** the person had reached that state of health and **what** the patient was now required to do to prevent a future event. The question, *Why me?* also often needed addressing. As well as giving the patient some answers, it could be helpful for the medical team as a clue to prevention.

> *"When something happens, particularly when it's out of the blue, the first question the person asks is:* Why me? *Cardiac rehabilitation and its education about the risk factors often give a very good clue as to why the patient has developed that particular condition in the first place. Not only is that helpful for the patients as it gives them answers, but it's also very helpful for the medical team because if you can track down why something's happened in the first place, you're much more likely to prevent it happening again."*

the journey begins

According to Dr Begg, the rehabilitation journey begins by looking at cardiac risk factors.

Whatever the reason for the patient presenting, cardiologists look at these **cardiac risk factors** that could include the patient having:

- a family history of heart disease
- associated high blood pressure
- diabetes
- habits such as smoking, lack of exercise, or poor eating choices.

"We concentrate on such factors when we're coordinating the program. The process is very much one of education, of making the patients aware of how they got there, where they are going, and what they can do to modify and improve their outcome.

"By educating the patients and empowering them and giving them confidence, it is much more likely they will avoid further complications. Such education will also improve their quality and quantity of life in the longer term.

"And there's plenty of evidence showing that people who undertake cardiac rehabilitation do better in the long term in relation to minimising further events and having a better quality of life – which is what it's all about."

downside

Unfortunately, there is a downside.

"One of the challenges of primary prevention (stopping the first event) is that people often are ***not receptive*** *to the educational, life-style-based, prevention message. Their* It won't happen to me *denial attitude doesn't help, either. Having had an event somewhat shatters that misconception, and the education messages suddenly become personally relevant."*

People who have had one cardiac event are at the highest risk of having another event. Despite this, the uptake of cardiac rehabilitation services around the world is relatively low. In Australia, it is only about 30 per cent.

JUDY'S EXPERIENCE

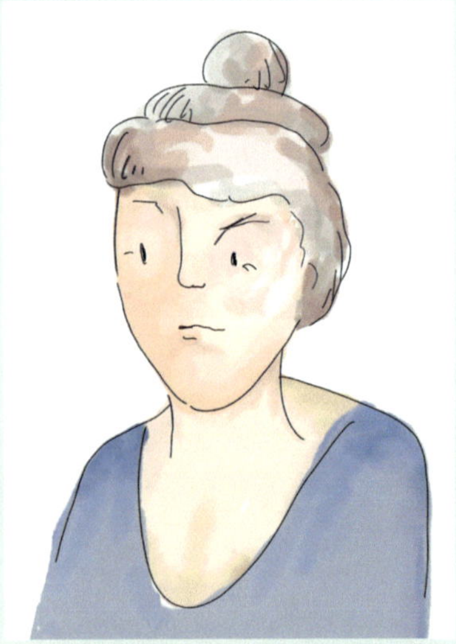

Judy was 70 years old when she came to see me (Warrick Bishop). She had had a heart attack about 10 years earlier. When we met, I saw a slim woman, casually dressed in jeans, sneakers, and a tee-shirt. I could smell cigarette smoke. She looked older than her stated years. The cigarettes had exacerbated a probable hard life, and I'm sure had contributed to her heart attack at a young age. Her referral asked me to assess her health as she hadn't seen a cardiologist during the 10 years since her heart attack.

As we started talking, it became very apparent very quickly that she was withdrawn, almost sullen, and she didn't like me. The temperature in the room dropped, and the atmosphere became most uncomfortable. After about 10 minutes, I had to be direct. I challenged her on her attitude and why she was at the appointment. After all, she had been referred to me, and she had come of her own volition. I said that it was tough to help someone who was so disengaged.

I gave her the option to go – Please go if you want to, and all the very best to you – *or stay* – Please stay if you want to. However, I can't help you while you won't talk to me.

Judy responded that she didn't like doctors.

I said that that was reasonable.

My experience shows that when people say they 'don't like doctors', they are really saying that they are afraid of what is associated with seeing a doctor.

After that, Judy loosened up a bit and engaged in the consultation, which meant that I had the opportunity to examine her history, look at current medications and her current medical condition. For a woman who was relatively young in this health scenario, she was limited in what she could do. Systematically, I prioritised a way forward, providing her general practitioner with a checklist of several different ideas to implement.

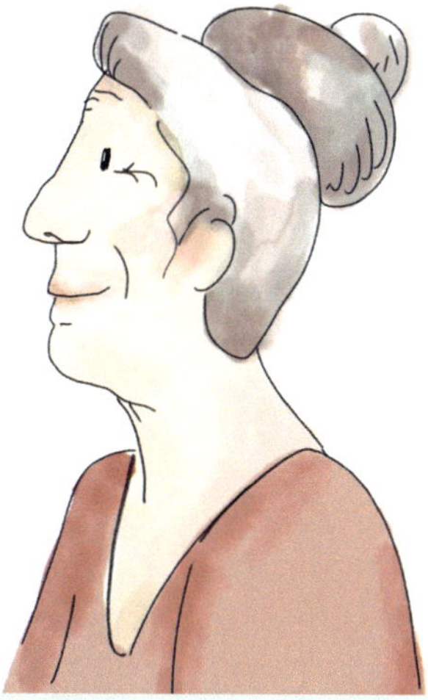

As Judy left, we shook hands. I wished her the best and invited her to keep in close contact with her general practitioner, who I knew was a good doctor who related well with patients and would follow through with the recommendations that I had made. I had spent longer than a standard consultation with Judy as I thought I would not see her again.

Walking into my waiting room several months later, I did a double take. There was Judy.

Me: What are you doing here?

Judy: You made me feel so well the last time Doc, I thought I'd come back and give you another go.

You need to look after your plumbing with the 3 Es

Cardiologist and author Dr Warrick Bishop speaks with cardiothoracic surgeon Dr Ashutosh Hardikar

who has a particular interest in cardiac rehabilitation, and is based at the Royal Hobart Hospital, Tasmania, Australia.

WB Ash, we've shared many patients over the years. Tell me, from a surgical perspective, why is cardiac rehabilitation important?

A *I think we both share a common belief that any intervention that you do as a cardiologist or me, as a cardiac surgeon, is a major step in a whole disease process that is unfolding. I genuinely believe that there has to be some kind of rehabilitation program where a person can adapt to a healthy lifestyle that can change the cardiovascular risk profile. And I think that is what got me into the cardiac rehab program.*

Any intervention we do as physicians is temporary; what I call, a glorified plumbing job, Warrick. It is what it is. It fixes the problem for the time being. ***Unless cardiac rehab becomes part of a patient's lifestyle in a long, sustained way, I don't think the fixing translates into a meaningful long-term change.***

WB What you are speaking about here is stopping people from having a second event, what is called secondary prevention. Each of us strongly believes that if someone has a first event, our obligation, our focus, is to try to reduce the chance of a second event occurring. So, secondary prevention is a huge component of rehabilitation. What are some of the factors within the provision of a rehab service you think are most important?

A *One thing people need to understand is that cardiac rehabilitation, generally, is an outpatient program based on the three Es: education, exercise, and emotional support.*

One E stands for education. It's quite vital that people get complete knowledge. A lot of our patients these days turn to Google and other search engines to find information, and that might not necessarily lead them to the most precise and the most scientifically accurate information. People need to have the right education about what the disease process is, what primary and secondary prevention mean, and what they can do, particularly in their personal context.

The second E is exercise. Unfortunately, that's all many people think rehabilitation is, an exercise regime. But it's a gradual program of, more importantly, what not to do as well. It's not just a set program that can be done from the internet. It is a personalised exercise program. So that's the second E.

And the third E is emotional support or counselling. And Warrick, I genuinely believe that the mental trauma that the cardiac surgery causes a patient, maybe subconsciously, is much more than the physical immobility I inflict on the patient. I think it's a scar on the mind. It's up to each individual. They can translate this to say: Oh, this is a game-changer in my life. This is a signal that I need to change my lifestyle and get back into healthy habits so that this does not happen again. I can improve my cardiovascular health.

WB I agree with you. I often use a car analogy when I speak to people about their heart and their heart's function. When it comes to an intervention like implanting a stent, or the need for bypass grafting, I say it's a bit like a car crash. We get to fix up the car pretty well, but sometimes we don't fix up the driver, and the driver is that mental change. It's a huge impost on people. I think it is part of a grieving process. The better we recognise that and help people through it, the smoother we can make that journey for them – and they're going to make that journey anyway.

A *Very nicely put, Warrick, very nicely put.*

I think that those are the essential components of it (based on) individualised planning. Each person is different. You know, some people are very well motivated, and some people need a lot of coaxing. We get a broad spectrum of patients, and we need a team of people involved to deliver this kind of program.

WB The emotional component, I think, is particularly interesting. I see a good number of patients who go through a near-death experience and then have a small wire cage inserted through the leg or the wrist to hold the artery open. These people are out of the hospital two days later. They barely missed a day in their lives. Yet, with cardiothoracic surgery, there's a substantial scar to remind them of what they have experienced. What do you think about the emotional impact between having a stent or bypass grafting (separate to the fact that we recognise one or the other would be used based on appropriate clinical grounds)?

A *I did my first cardiac surgery in 1994, so I can say that over the years, I've seen a lot of people go through both stents and surgery, in India, the UK, and Australia. Nine times out of 10, people would choose a stent, just for this emotional apprehension. Besides, no-one likes the physical trauma of surgery, to be 'cut open' as they put it. You know, people have some gruesome concepts about cardiac surgeries because they watch videos or famous television programs. And it might not necessarily be the best thing for a lot of people because that keeps more emotional and mental images and scars rather than educating them about the process. And look, when I get old, the first thing even I'm going to ask is, "Is this fixable by a stent?" It's a natural question for people to ask, and it's not just the physical part of it. I think there is a lot of mental scarring. So, the emotional reaction to it is what creates a lot of trauma.*

WB When faced with the need for a procedure, people choose the most straightforward path available to them, and we try to facilitate that option. The desire – and the necessity – to change is higher in the patients who have gone through the harder journey. I see people who breeze in, have a stent implanted, don't realise they have nearly died, and don't embrace the change that they should because they think, *Oh, that was so easy, I won't worry about it!*

A *Sure. A well-made point. The morbidity of surgery, the pain, and the scars remind people that the surgical wounds take time to heal. Usually, four to six weeks are needed before the breastbone heals, and people can start driving, and many people take a few weeks to get back into independent, daily living activities. So, it is a reminder,*

I think, for all of us that the more time we have to spend with an ailment reinforces those brain circuits which tell us, Hey, you need to change (your behaviour) otherwise this is what you have to go through.

You know, when people come for surgery, they are looking for longevity as well because they don't want to go through this again. And, as you know, probably the only place where surgery scores over stents is in multi-vessel coronary artery disease. Surgery promises to offer a better long-term result, albeit, with a bit more short-term pain. So, you know, no gain without pain is true – and especially true in our field.

WB Perhaps we should bind up our stent patients with a constricting thoracic bandage for a couple of weeks so that they have the impression of the significance of it all!

Ash, you have had the experience of setting up a rehabilitation unit in India. There were some aspects that you thought were valuable, yet we are not replicating them here, in Australia. Would you like to speak to that?

A *I started a unit in India in 2001 when I went back after formal training at the Royal Adelaide Hospital (South Australia). Although I had seen the Australian program, I was most impressed by what a friend of mine showed me at the Singapore University Hospital. It has one of the very dedicated cardiac rehabilitation units built on a team approach. The team had:*

- *a medical doctor who was a cardiologist with a particular interest in rehabilitation*
- *a nursing coordinator*
- *an educator, also a nurse*
- *a dietician*
- *a physiotherapist*
- *an occupational therapist*
- *psychologists and*
- *exercise specialists.*

They had a separate building and the unit attracted large numbers of patients.

I was just so impressed by the way they could influence change. I mean, people had a variety of problems: might be psychosocial, might be how to get back to work, some people had some physical ailments which didn't allow them certain exercises, and there were exercise consultants. But more importantly I thought, there was a cardiologist involved who had a very clear idea of secondary prevention goals. He knew a particular patient's targets.

I feel the difference in Australia, because everything is Medicare-funded, is that the funding for the programs never matches the need. We cannot stress enough that cardiovascular disease, such as heart and stroke events, are responsible for more than one-third of the deaths in the adult Australian population, and yet, the importance we give this program is not the same. While not all cardiologists will be dedicated to long-term secondary prevention because that might not be their primary interest, we need to have a spirit of keeping people as well as possible for as long as possible and the data is clear in preventing recurring heart problems, so let's do it.

If we were to have a mechanism and a team of people to reiterate to these 25,000 people before or after their intervention, that, Guys watch out; this is what you need to do; this is the healthy lifestyle for you, *I think Hobart would lose the country's top-ranking as the capital for cardiovascular disease. We would be able to improve. So, I think there is a lack of having a complete expert team, in one facility, in one place. And more importantly, a clinician, a rehab nurse, the physio or exercise physiologist and dietician could all work together for the best outcome of the patient.*

WB How often should we re-engage with people during their ongoing journey? Once the person has gone through rehab, do we see them six-monthly, 12-monthly, two-yearly, five-yearly? There's no question that, as humans, we all drift back to our initial habits. So, would 12 months be your preferred interval between visits for following up for these post-intervention rehabilitation cases?

A *That would be the minimum. And as you know, there would be some people who might need more support, because they're isolated in the community, or because they have some kind of special need.*

Let's say, some people find it really hard to give up smoking. Quitting requires a genuine psychological intervention that has to be done gently, and they might need more frequent visits. And you might need a smoking cessation nurse as a part of that program, keeping the original cardiologist in the loop.

WB As we finish, I invite you to share one of your many patient stories.

A *Absolutely. I can share a story about a lovely guy and his wife from the eastern coast of Tasmania. He came for second-time valve surgery. As you know, each operation can be with complications, and unfortunately, and this time, his heart did not respond well. This guy had to go on artificial heart-lung machine support – ECMO or extracorporeal membrane oxygenation – for seven to eight days.*

Luckily, and his angels were looking after him, he responded well. On the eighth day, he came off that artificial life support. It took him two weeks to get out of ICU and then he spent another week in the ward before joining a rehabilitation program, which became very important to his recovery.

One of his drugs caused a side-effect which produced Parkinson-like symptoms for quite a time, and he was mentally really, really down. He had an extremely supportive wife, and they moved into a Hobart suburb where they rented a place so he could attend the rehab program.

Eight weeks down the line when I met him, again, he was a changed person, Warrick. The rehab experience had taken away the negativity that the traumatic experience had created in his mind, and he was able to get over the scars. He was able to say, This is a new lease to my life. *He said the rehabilitation really helped him to start again. The experience is somewhat like a child learning to walk. He had overcome the Parkinson's symptoms, and his heart was looking a lot better.*

*So, I get a call at Easter time saying that he is out in the garden, and the wife says they all are thankful for the team. And that's where I thought, **"If that rehab team was not there, my plumbing job has no meaning."** You see, it has to be a complete unit that delivers. In this man's case, it was not just the exercise specialist. It was also the psychologist who got through to him and the occupational therapist who made small changes at his home so that he could gently get back into walking and doing things. So, it was really, really good.*

WB How satisfying to see someone in such a difficult situation to get a life back and have a quality of life again.

A *Absolutely.*

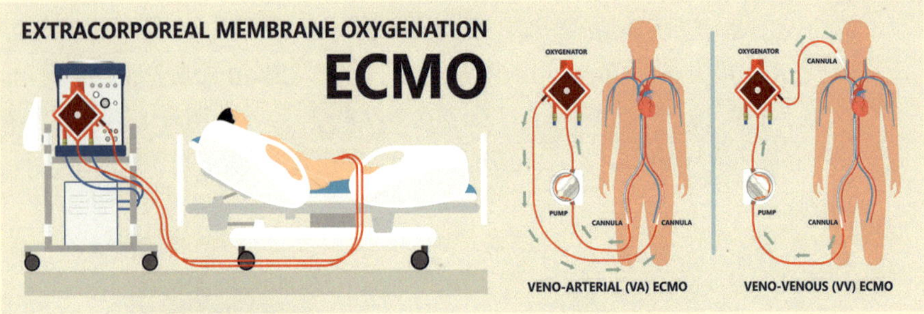

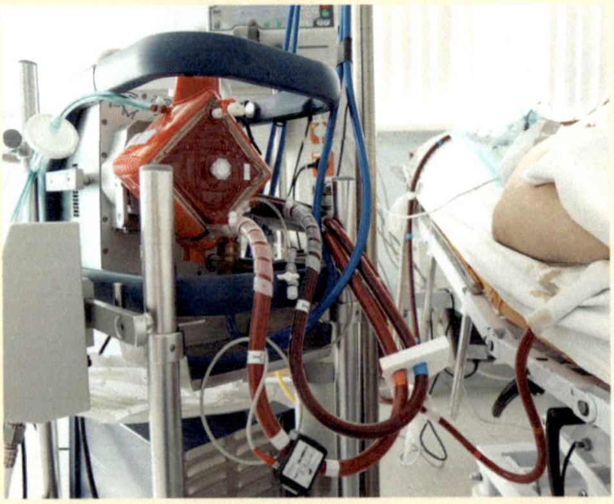

What ECMO means is that the person's blood leaves the body and is treated in a machine that acts as the heart and lungs outside of the body. The blood then gets pumped back into the body to complete the circulation. ECMO is an extraordinary piece of life-saving technology.

understanding ECMO

WB Some final words?

A *Everyone is getting more evidence-based. There is a famous review system called the Cochrane Reviews. In 2011[10], they came up with what we call a meta-analysis[11] in which they looked at thousands of published articles in this field. And they very clearly showed that cardiac rehabilitation has a mortality benefit as well. And that mortality benefit is very clear across the studies, across different continents. So, a program like this with the three Es that we talked to, exercise, education, and the emotional support, will not only help regain strength, but it also prevents worsening or recurrences, and* ***improves both the quality and quantity of the patient's life.***

WB There's no question that if we do those three Es, well, we're investing a small amount to save a lot down the line. *(ASH, Absolutely.)* Plus, we're getting incredible dividends.

ASH'S STORY – As a kid in India, I read in Reader's Digest about a famous cardiac surgeon in the United Kingdom and became very inspired. My father was a schoolteacher. He had a lot of students who were the children of doctors go through, and I looked up to doctors as people who could contribute in a different way to society. But that particular series on the cardiac surgeon, Sir Magdi Yacoub, inspired me. So, right from my childhood days, I was pretty sure what I wanted to be.

IMPORTANT POINTS

- A cardiac event is rarely a planned occurrence in a person's life – and help is needed.
- Cardiovascular disease (CVD) is the most common cause of death in the world.
- Cardiac rehabilitation is a journey that supports people to live life as well as possible for as long as possible after a cardiac diagnosis or event.
- Cardiac rehab benefits include
  - living longer
  - improved functional capacity
  - better quality of life
  - fewer hospital readmissions.
- Cardiac rehab is one of the most clinically and cost-effective therapeutic interventions in CVD management.
- Cardiac rehab uptake, worldwide, is poor.

---

1 *World Economic Forum, "As the COVID-19 death toll pass 1 million, how does it compare to other major killers?" https://www.weforum.org/agenda/2020/09/covid-19-deaths-global-killers-comparison/*

2 *Dr Alistair Begg, rehabilitation cardiologist, Adelaide, South Australia, Australia, speaking in a podcast interview with Dr Warrick Bishop, cardiologist, Hobart, Tasmania, Australia, for the Healthy Heart Network: www.healthyheartnetwork.com podcast episodes 119, 120 and 121.*

3 *World Economic Forum, "As the COVID-19 death toll pass 1 million, how does it compare to other major killers?" https://www.weforum.org/agenda/2020/09/covid-19-deaths-global-killers-comparison/ CVD is well ahead of cancer, which claimed 9.5 million lives world-wide, and respiratory disease – 3.91 million*

4 *World Health Organization website https://www.who.int/health-topics/cardiovascular-diseases#tab=tab_1*

5 *According to the Australian Institute of Health Welfare, CVD was the underlying cause of death in 41,800 Australian deaths (26% of all deaths) and an associated cause in 70,600 deaths, in 2018.*

6 *The World Heart Federation defines secondary cardiovascular prevention as any strategy aimed to reduce the probability of a recurrent cardiovascular event in patients with atherosclerotic cardiovascular disease, including coronary artery disease, cerebrovascular artery disease, peripheral artery disease, and atherosclerotic aortic disease. https://www.world-heart-federation.org/cvd-roadmaps/whf-global-roadmaps/secondary-prevention/*

7 *Anderson L, Thompson DR, Oldridge N, Zwisler A, Rees K, Martin N, Taylor RS. Exercise-based cardiac rehabilitation of coronary heart disease. Cochrane Database of Systematic Reviews. 2016; Issue 1(Art. No.: CD001800.) Available at: http://onlinelibrary.wiley.com/doi/10.1002/14651858.CD001800.pub3/abstract*

8 *World Health Organization. Needs and action priorities in cardiac rehabilitation and secondary prevention in patients with CHD. Geneva World Health Organization. Available from http://whqlibdoc.who.int/euro/- 1993/EUR_ICP_CVD_125.pdf 1993*

9 *Healthy Heart Network (www.healthyheartnetwork.com) podcast episodes 119, 120 and 121. All quotes by Dr Begg in this chapter are from the same podcast interview.*

10 *The 2011 work was updated in 2021: https://www.cochrane.org/CD001800/VASC_exercise-based-rehabilitation-coronary-heart-disease*

11 *If the results of the individual studies are combined to produce an overall statistic, this is usually called a meta-analysis. Many Cochrane Reviews measure benefits and harms by collecting data from more than one trial and combining them to generate an average result. This aims to provide a more precise estimate of the effects of an intervention and to reduce uncertainty. A systematic review attempts to identify, appraise, and synthesise all the empirical evidence that meets pre-specified eligibility criteria to answer a specific research question. Researchers conducting systematic reviews use explicit, systematic methods that are selected with a view aimed at minimising bias, to produce more reliable findings to inform decision making. Cochrane Library. https://www.cochranelibrary.com/about/about-cochrane-reviews*

Before delving too far into rehab programs, let us look more closely at the heart, what makes it 'tick', and what can go wrong. Let's understand better how the heart functions.

GETTING BACK TO BASICS

UNDERSTANDING THE HEART

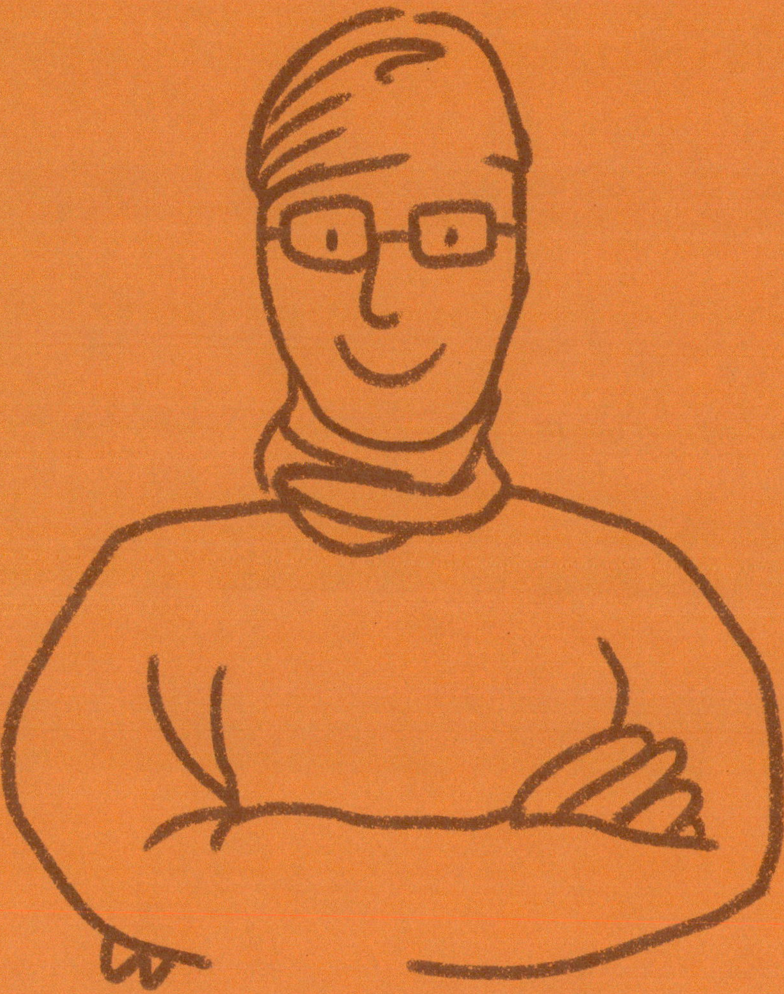

chapter 2

A FINELY TUNED PUMP

When most people think of problems with the heart, their immediate thought is 'heart attack'. Their instant image is what they have seen in the movies or on television, of the guy clutching his chest, passing out and falling to the floor. This is the classic 'heart attack'; someone has a blockage in an artery that causes chest pain. The lack of blood flow may lead to cardiac rhythm disturbance that causes the person to pass out when the heart stops beating (cardiac arrest). Interestingly, 'heart attack' is not a medical term. Rather, it is a lay term reserved mainly for a blockage in the artery that causes damage or death to at least some part of the heart muscle. For about one in 20 people, not only does the heart muscle die, so does the person[12]. Blocked arteries are not the only cause of a 'heart attack'. Trouble with the heart's rhythm or the heart's pumping capacity can also trigger problems for the heart.

To better understand this, let's look at the heart and how it functions.

Essentially, **the heart is a large muscle that pumps blood** through our bodies. The **blood** supplies nutrients and oxygen **to** the body and removes waste such as carbon dioxide **from** the body. The muscle of the heart is the first organ in the body to receive blood after it enters the aorta from the left ventricle.

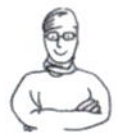

A well-functioning heart contracts rhythmically, pumping blood to the body roughly 100,000 times a day, which is about 35 million times a year and over three billion times in a lifetime!

The heart can be likened to a car engine. It has

- an **engine block** that generates the power
  - *the muscle of the heart, the* myocardium (myo, *muscle;* cardium, *of the heart)*
- with its **pistons** (compression chambers) and **valves**
  - *the heart is a four-chambered structure, with two chambers on the right-hand side and two chambers on the left-hand side. On each side, there is a pre-pumping chamber, the atrium, which is joined to a main pumping chamber, the ventricle.*

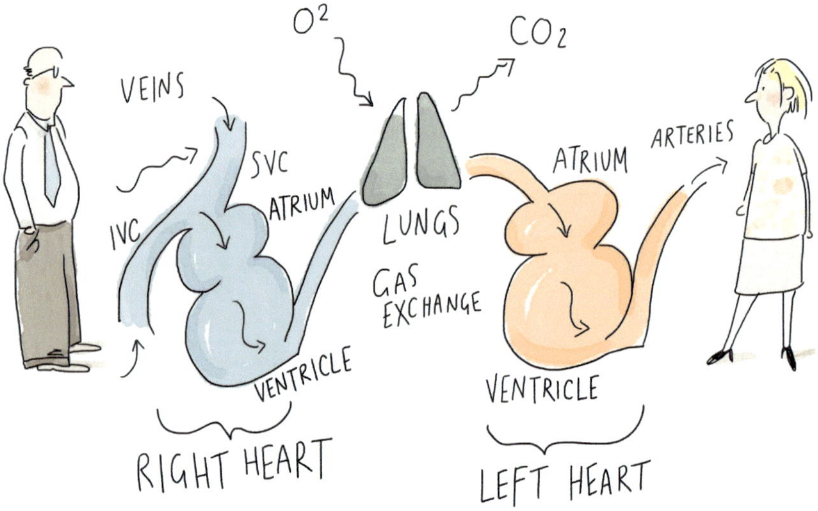

a schematic showing the flow of the blood from the veins through the heart to the arteries

  - *this means the heart has two pumps*
    > *there is a right atrium and ventricle combination that receives the carbon dioxide-rich blood from the body and pumps it to the lungs for the carbon dioxide/oxygen exchange and*

    > *there is a left atrium-ventricle combination that pumps the oxygen-rich blood from the lungs into the body. The left ventricle (LV) is the main pumping chamber of the heart.*

- *they are the 'right heart' and the 'left heart', respectively. The sides pump together with each atrium contracting marginally ahead of its ventricle. From the LV the blood flows into the aorta and then around the body.*
- *several strategically placed valves stop the blood flowing in the wrong direction. Healthy valves are important for good heart function, maximising pump efficiency so the heart can function throughout a lifetime. Each time the heart beats valves open and close to allow the blood to flow.*

- an **electrical system**
  - *which, in the heart, ensures synchronicity and coordinated contraction within the four chambers and also has a mechanism for acceleration and deceleration.*
- a set of **fuel lines** supplying the cylinders of the car
  - *the coronary arteries arise from the aorta and are the first branches in the body's circulatory system: the right coronary artery and the left main coronary artery (which divides into the left anterior descending artery, and the circumflex artery).*
  - *these major arteries comprise less than 35 cm in total length and less than 5 mm in diameter at the largest site. A single build-up of plaque leading to a blockage may only be 1 cm in length. This is a very vulnerable system.*

A problem with the heart can be caused by a blocked fuel line (artery) or 'rust in the pipes', the electrical system playing up, or a problem with the pistons and valves.

A CLOSER LOOK

flow of blood through the heart and the lungs

Blood flows from the body to the heart through the veins, collecting into two major veins called the **superior vena cava** (SVC) ① *(refer to the diagram on the facing page)* and the **inferior vena cava** (IVC) ① which drain into the right side of the heart.

This oxygen-poor, dark purple, carbon dioxide-rich blood arrives in the **right atrium** ② where it receives a gentle pump through the **tricuspid valve**, a one-way valve, into the **right ventricle** ③.

The ventricle then pumps the blood through another one-way valve, the **pulmonary valve**, into the lungs, via the **pulmonary artery** ④ ⑤.

Within the lungs, **gas exchange occurs**; the air we breathe in provides oxygen and the breath we exhale carries away carbon dioxide. The blood becomes replenished with fresh oxygen for use by the body.

Bright red, oxygen-rich arterial blood then flows from the lungs through the **four pulmonary veins** ⑥ to the **left atrium** ⑦.

The left atrium gives a gentle pump and the blood passes through the **mitral valve**, another one-way valve, into the **left ventricle** ⑧.

The left ventricle then contracts, squeezing blood through the **aortic valve**, another one-way valve, into the main artery of the body, the **aorta** ⑨ ⑩, to begin its journey around the body.

The left ventricle is the main pumping chamber of the heart.

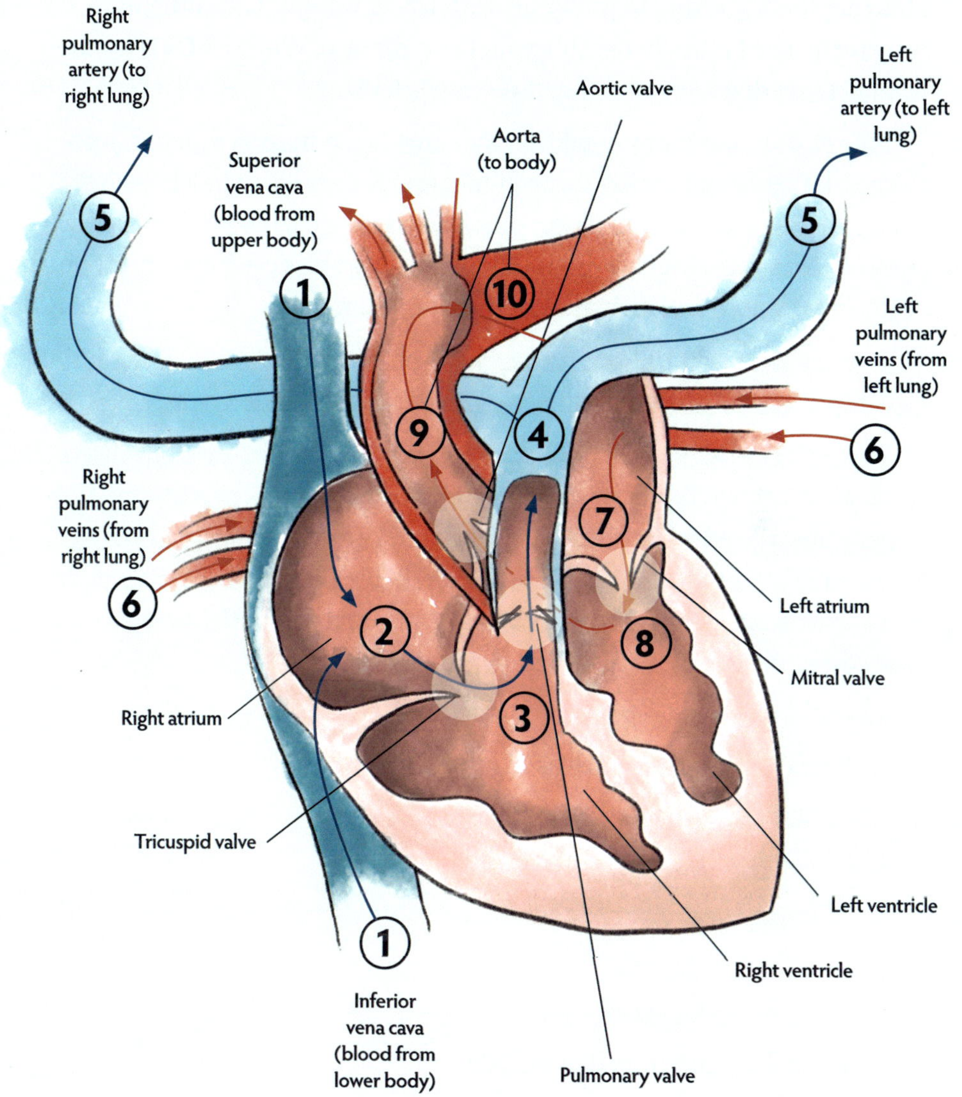

blood flow and connections inside the heart

heart disease

Cardiovascular disease (CVD) is the umbrella term for all diseases affecting the heart due to problems with blood vessels. Often the term is incorrectly used interchangeably with heart disease. While all CVD can be termed heart disease, not all heart disease is CVD.

Heart disease is any condition that affects the normal functioning of the heart. Conditions include congenital heart defects (such as a hole in the heart), diseases affecting the heart muscle, blockages to the arteries such as coronary artery disease that causes heart attack, problems with the function of the heart valves and arrhythmias (heart rhythm).

Studies show that about 50 per cent of heart disease is caused by hereditary factors; the other 50 per cent relates to lifestyle issues.

Hereditary factors include family history, such as a 'first-degree' relative (biological mother, father or sibling) having heart disease, particularly if it is early onset (under 55 years of age for males and under 60 years of age for females). Family history is a non-modifiable risk factor. Age, gender and ethnicity are other **non-modifiable** risk factors for the presence of heart disease.

Lifestyle influences include

- behavioural factors such as
  - smoking
  - eating a poor diet
  - being overweight or obese
  - failing to exercise
  - living under stress, and
- physiological factors that include
  - high blood pressure (hypertension)
  - worsening cholesterol profile, and
  - high blood sugars.

These lifestyle factors are **modifiable**, or **reversible**, risk factors linked to underlying social determinants such as life choices, income and urbanisation, and they are a focus in cardiac rehabilitation.

A person's prognosis improves through bringing more factors under control, giving the person a better chance of surviving 10, 15, 20 years after the heart event.

Then, there are patients who have no clear family history and who seem to be looking after themselves. They are not overweight; they don't smoke. They exercise and eat a healthy diet. They have not developed diabetes, nor do they have high blood pressure or cholesterol issues. Yet, despite seemingly to have done everything 'right', they still find themselves with a heart problem. (Remember Ron from our Introduction?)

IMPORTANT POINTS ✓

- The heart is a large muscle that pumps blood through our bodies.
- The heart can be likened to a car engine. It has an
    - engine block that generates the power (the muscle of the heart)
        - > with its pistons (compression chambers – the atria and ventricles) and
        - > valves
    - an electrical system
    - a set of fuel lines (coronary arteries) supplying the cylinders of the car.
- Heart disease can involve
    - hereditary factors which are non-modifiable risk factors and
    - lifestyle behavioural and/or physiological factors which are modifiable

12 *Heart Foundation website: https://www.heartfoundation.org.au/Activities-finding-or-opinion/key-statistics-heart-attack This equates to one person dying of a heart attack every 74 minutes, or on average 19 people every day, in Australia.*

The heart's electrical system coordinates a powerful pump.

chapter 3

AN ELECTRICAL MASTERPIECE

A healthy heart is a highly efficient pump coordinated by its electrical system. The atria and ventricles work together, alternately contracting and relaxing to pump blood through the heart and into the body. The heartbeat is triggered by electrical impulses. The heart pumps three to four litres of blood every minute, with the healthy heart rate between 50 and 100 beats per minute.

Normally, the contractions of the atria are set off by the heart's natural pacemaker, a small area of the heart called the **sinoatrial (SA) node**, located in the top of the right atrium. This is where the electrical activity 'beats the drum' to which the rest of the heart 'marches'.

Electrical impulses travel rapidly throughout the atria, a bit like a Mexican wave, causing the muscle fibres to contract, squeezing blood into the ventricles. To reach the ventricles, these electrical impulses pass through the **atrioventricular (AV) node**, a cluster of cells in the centre of the heart, between the atria and the ventricles. This node acts as a gatekeeper. Passing through this node **slows** the electrical impulses before they enter the ventricles, thus giving the atria time to contract before the ventricles then contract. Once in the ventricles, the electrical impulse is carried via special cells, **Purkinje fibres**, which act like wires delivering the signal to the apex of the heart, ensuring that blood is expelled from the furthest point first.

When the electrical system of the heart goes wrong, the heart beats out of rhythm. The rate of the heartbeat and/or its regularity can be affected.

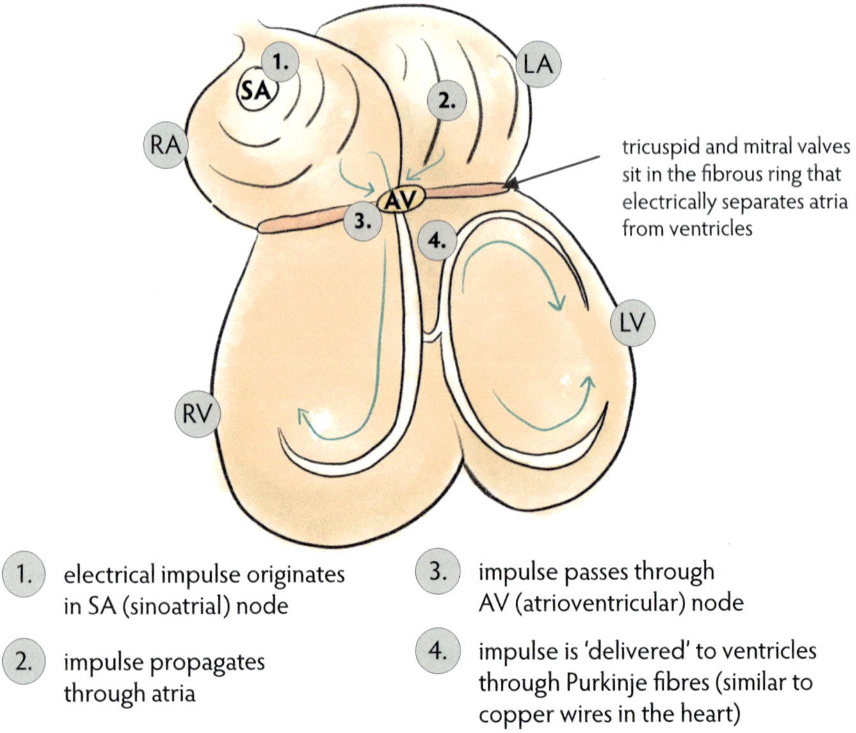

the electrical system

atrial fibrillation

The most common heart arrhythmia presenting to hospitals and cardiologists is atrial fibrillation (AF), a condition in which the heartbeat is 'irregularly irregular'. Often felt as a sudden, rapid, irregular and chaotic heartbeat, this common heart rhythm problem can also be present without the patient experiencing any symptoms. The impact of the condition on the patient ranges from inconvenience to black out, to chest pain and heart failure, with stroke another potential and devastating complication.

More than 33.5 million people worldwide, or 0.5 per cent of the world's population, have the condition[13] and this rises to 15-20 per cent of people over the age of 80. These figures make AF a serious global health problem, and one that is increasing significantly each year. While AF can be managed, at this time[14] there is no cure.

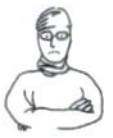

AF is the most common presentation to cardiologists, and it has overtaken heart attacks and heart failure as the most common presentation to hospitals. It is the tsunami of cardiac disease in our time.

AF occurs when electrical impulses in the atria, the upper chambers of the heart, become chaotic, and instead of producing a steady, regular beat, they generate a scattered irregular, very fast and uncontrolled heartbeat. These chaotic impulses from the atria transmit to the main pumping chambers, the ventricles, and that beat, too, becomes irregularly irregular. As a result, the heart does not pump properly.

People often present with the classic symptom of palpitation which can be accompanied by a range of indicators including lack of energy, breathlessness, dizziness, chest tightness, poor appetite, swelling of the ankles. When the heart doesn't pump well, blood can stagnate in the left atrium, in the left atrial appendage, and clot. If the clot breaks away and travels to the brain, it causes a stroke.

Unfortunately, while it is an increasingly common condition, many people are unaware of having it as AF can be asymptomatic – and found as an incidental finding (when the patient is undergoing a health check or is being treated for another condition) or when the person presents with a devastating stroke. **Too late.**

Other rhythm disturbances are atrial ectopic beats and ventricular ectopic beats (extra beats in either the atria or the ventricles), atrial flutter (similar to AF), supraventricular tachycardia (fast beats arising above the ventricles), ventricular tachycardia (rapid rhythm arising in the ventricle), ventricular fibrillation (chaotic rhythm in the ventricle that is not felt by the person; it is not life-sustaining, and the most likely cause of sudden cardiac death).

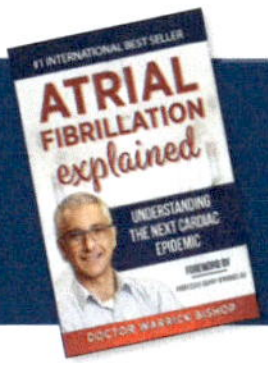

For further information on atrial fibrillation, please see Appendix 3 and Dr Bishop's book, *Atrial Fibrillation Explained* (page 295 for details)

IMPORTANT POINTS

- When the electrical system of the heart malfunctions, the heart beats out of rhythm, affecting the pump action of the heart. This is called arrhythmia.
- The heartbeat and/or its regularity can be affected so the heart beats too fast, too slow and/or irregularly.
- While there are several possible heart arrhythmias, atrial fibrillation's (AF) 'irregularly irregular' or chaotic rhythm is one of the most common, with the serious complication of stroke.
- AF is a manageable condition, but it cannot be cured.

---

13 *World Health Organisation study: Atrial Fibrillation is a growing global health concern, https://www.cedars-sinai.org/newsroom/world-health-organization-study-atrial-fibrillation-is-a-growing-global-health-concern/*

14 *2022*

Our coronary arteries, the fuel lines of the body, are at the heart of the matter when it comes to a heart attack.

chapter 4

THE 'HEART' OF THE MATTER

The all-important coronary arteries, the fuel lines of our car analogy, are not only the beginning of the body's circulatory system, but they are also 'at the heart' of a heart attack.

We have already mentioned the flow of blood through the heart and lungs for the carbon dioxide-oxygen exchange. As the oxygen-rich blood, our fuel, leaves the left ventricle via the aorta for its life-giving journey around the body, it travels initially through the coronary arteries which are the first branches in the circulatory system. The heart itself is the first organ to receive blood.

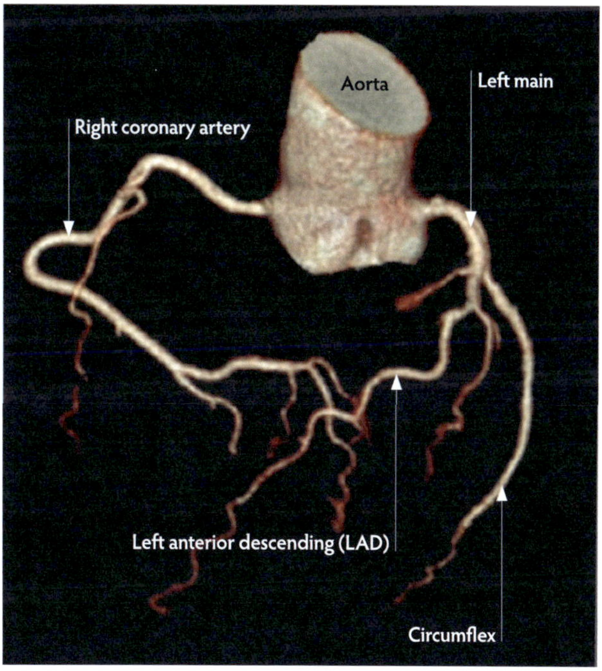

the coronary tree as seen on cardiac CT imaging

This system consists of the **left main coronary artery** and the **right coronary artery**. Within one centimetre the **left main coronary artery** divides into two arteries:

- the **left anterior descending artery** which provides blood to the anterior surface of the heart, which is the surface nearest the chest wall, and
- the **circumflex artery** which supplies blood to the back of the heart, which is the surface of the heart nearest the spine.

The **right coronary artery** supplies the inferior surface of the heart, which is the surface that is nearest the diaphragm.

The terms 'right dominant' or 'left dominant' are used in reference to the artery that supplies blood to the bulk of the inferior surface of the heart (the surface nearest the diaphragm). This is usually from the right coronary artery and, therefore, termed 'right dominant'. Sometimes, however, the right coronary artery is smaller and the circumflex artery (the one that branches off the left main coronary artery and wraps around the heart) is bigger, or 'dominant'. When the left coronary artery supplies the majority of the inferior surface of the heart, it is called 'left dominant'.

Size becomes significant in terms of the amount of the heart that may be affected by a blockage of the artery, the dominant artery providing blood to a larger territory.

Most often, the left anterior descending artery is the largest and most important of the three main coronary arteries. It can be 12 to 14cm long while only two to five millimetres in diameter. This dimension is a little thicker than a pen refill, yet its blockage can be disastrous. A dominant right coronary artery can be approximately the same size and a non-dominant circumflex can be six to eight centimetres long and 1.5 to three millimetres in diameter. The major arteries are comprised of fewer than 35cm in total length and fewer than five millimetres in diameter at their largest.

coronary artery disease

At a cellular level, wear and tear and stress combined with inflammation in the artery can cause 'rusting of the pipes' or plaque development within the artery, which can lead to **coronary artery disease** (CAD).[15]

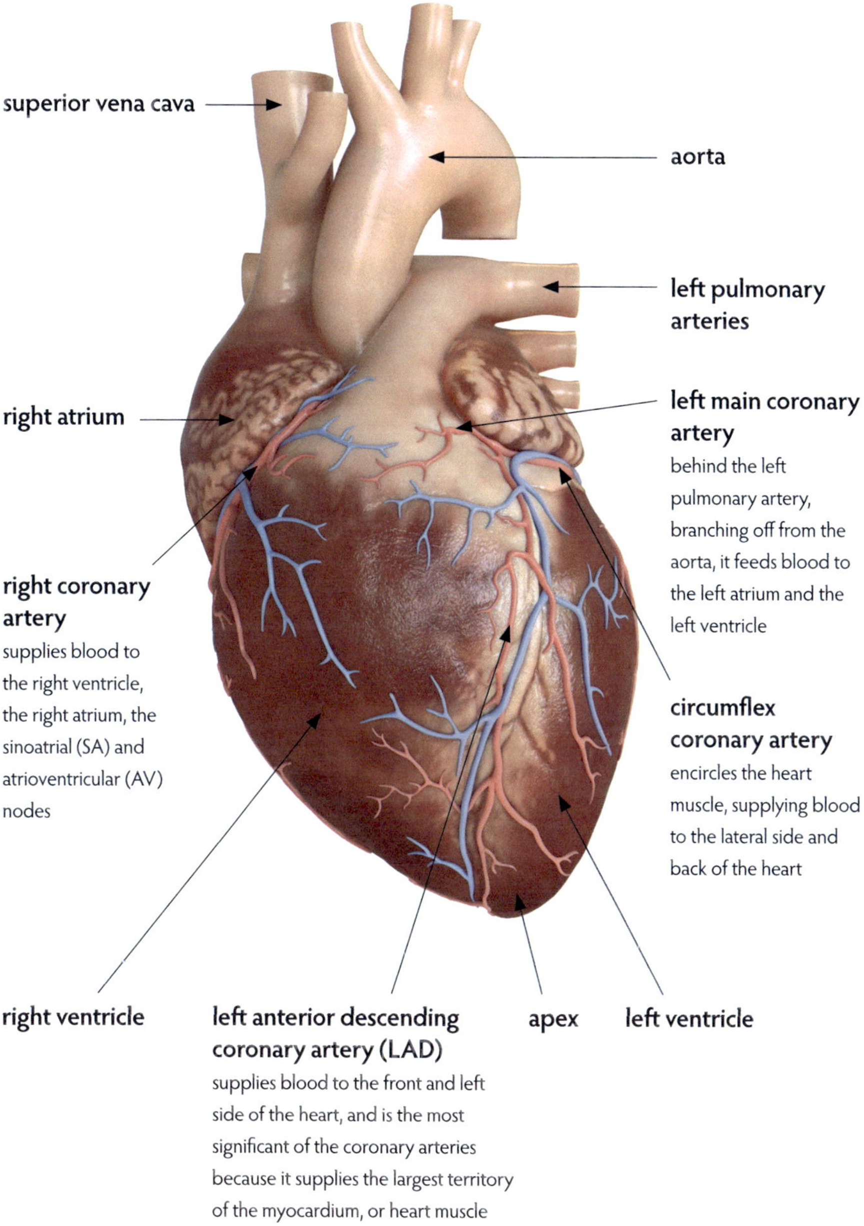

In this diagram, the coronary arteries are pink and cardiac veins are blue. Cardiac veins carry the de-oxygenated blood from the myocardium (heart muscle) to the right atrium so it can be sent to the lungs for re-oxygenation.

CAD is the process of atherosclerosis, or plaque, build-up in the arteries that leads to impaired blood flow causing symptoms or loss of function.

Certain areas inside the arteries are more prone to this type of wear and tear, especially where there are high-flow and shear stresses. The start of the left anterior descending (LAD) artery, the main artery down the front of the heart, is a very common spot for plaque build-up.

Wear and tear on arteries may be related to the very specific twists and turns and the path that the artery takes over the heart, keeping in mind that the heart is constantly moving underneath it. There is no way to evaluate that wear and tear, at least in the current era. And so, occasionally, a heart problem occurs in people who appear to be healthy and at low risk.

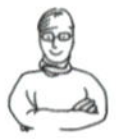

The wear and tear problem is a complicated area where research is being undertaken, and it reminds us that we don't fully understand everything to do with coronary artery disease.

patchy process

At best, coronary artery disease is a patchy process. Autopsies have shown that generally a focal (localised area) lesion (plaque) has led to the life ending event. Within the same artery, there can be areas that may not be diseased to the same extent, or even at all. And the plaque build-up can be flow-limiting or non-flow-limiting.

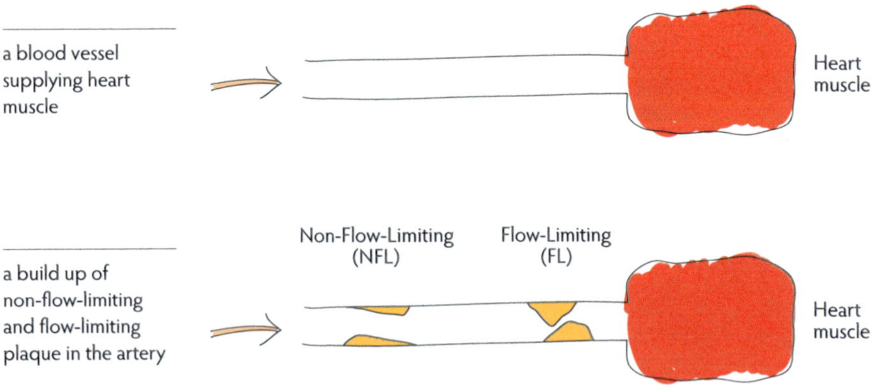

Autopsies after sudden cardiac death from coronary artery disease show that up to 60 per cent of the culprit lesions were flow-limiting, or tight, prior to the event that led to death and, hence, likely to have given a clue by way of chest pain or shortness of breath.

This leaves about 40 per cent that had been non-flow-limiting before the event. Here, the person has no warning, no symptoms. The event – even death – strikes suddenly. Often, the person appears to be fit and healthy.

Similar components are found in both flow-limiting and non-flow-limiting lesions:

- the wall of the artery;
- the lumen (or inside space) of the artery;
- the cholesterol plaque which has built-up and is beginning to intrude into the artery, and
- a fibrous cap that separates the plaque contents from the blood.

The blood contains many components. Importantly, there are platelets, those small particles responsible for the formation of a clot when an abnormality is detected with the inside lining of the artery.

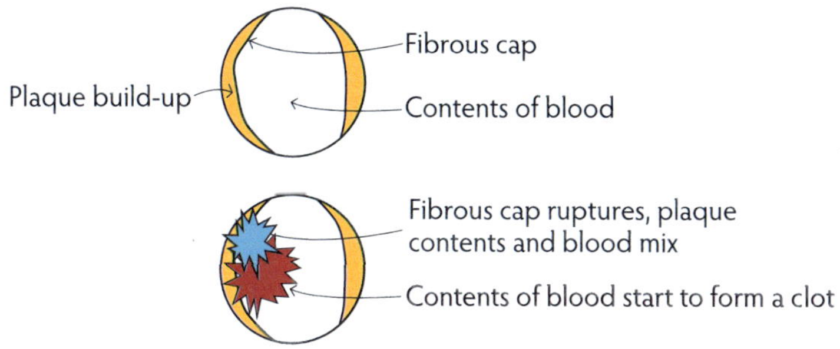

a schematic showing how, when the contents of the plaque come into contact with the contents of the blood, the body begins to form a clot

Should the fibrous covering of the build-up of cholesterol rupture, the blood encounters the contents of the plaque. The platelets, having rapidly detected the change, start to come together to form a clot which may progress to a complete blockage of the artery. Even a microscopic tear in the fibrous cap can lead to the formation of a clot, which can then rapidly block off that artery and be life-ending.

Ten to 15 per cent of people who suffer a heart attack die[16], and many receive no warning.

In the right setting, the formation of a clot is a very good thing. When we suffer a cut, the platelets clump at the site of the wound and save us from bleeding to death.

historically

Historically, the first time that a problem with the arteries could be suspected was when symptoms presented:

- **angina** – discomfort in the chest when pain is experienced in association with exertion (the term has its root meaning in a sense of strangulation);
- **shortness of breath** on exertion – can indicate a lack of blood flowing to the heart,

or

- an **acute coronary syndrome** – the sudden development of a complete, or near complete, blockage of a coronary artery. A lessened blood flow to a region of the heart muscle results in damage. A complete blockage causes the death of that area of the heart muscle. This is our 'heart attack' or, medically, a **myocardial infarction** (*myo*, muscle, *cardio*, heart, *infarction*, death by lack of blood flow). A near complete blockage, or **unstable angina**, puts stress on the heart and can be a forerunner to a complete blockage.

Please, please, please seek medical help should you be affected by chest pain or unexplained shortness of breath.

cardiac CT imaging

Although detection and treatment of coronary artery disease, historically, has been related to the presence of symptoms or the occurrence of a major coronary event, rapid improvements and ongoing development in cardiac CT imaging are making this less the case.

The CT imaging offers precise information around the health of an individual's arteries.

There are two groups of patients who may be considered for CT imaging of the heart. The first group is **symptomatic** patients for whom imaging would be used for evaluation of possible narrowing of the arteries. The second group consists of **asymptomatic** patients and CT imaging would be used for risk evaluation[17] – literally looking at the health of the arteries before a problem occurs. *(further detail, page 67)*

what is plaque?

The build-up of cholesterol, scavenger cells, scar tissue and calcium in the wall of the artery is called **atherosclerotic plaque**, or for ease of expression, plaque.

To understand this better, let's look at the parts of the artery.

The arteries are made up of three layers: the inner layer (*tunica intima*, meaning inner coat), the middle layer (*tunica media*, middle coat), and the outer layer (*tunica adventitia*, outside coat).

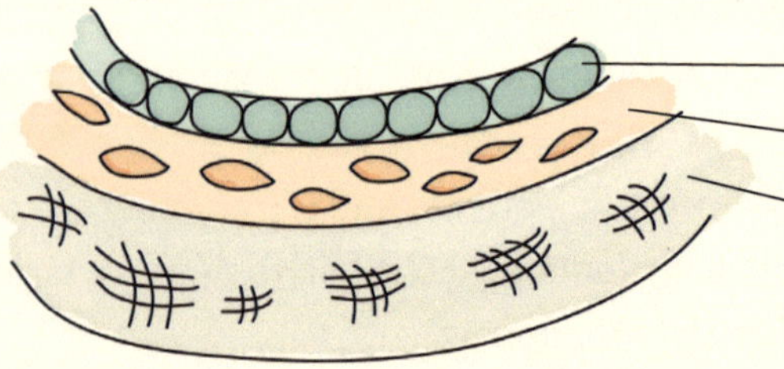

The **inner layer** is a smooth lining made from **endothelial cells** (*endo*, inside, and *thelium*, skin). This inner layer, or endothelium, ensures that the blood runs smoothly through the blood vessel and does not stick to the wall of the artery. It also responds to stresses and strains within the artery and then communicates with the muscle layer to influence relaxation and contraction.

The **middle layer** is made up predominantly of special **muscle cells** called smooth muscle. They are different to the muscles in your legs which are skeletal muscle, or, in your heart, which are cardiac muscle. Smooth muscles are not controlled by nerves in the way the skeletal muscles are. Instead, they respond to the automatic regulatory systems of the body. As the smooth muscle contracts, it narrows the arteries. As the same amount of blood is being pumped through a narrower blood vessel, blood pressure increases. (This is oversimplified but it relates the basic idea.) So, this layer of the blood vessel has a significant influence on blood pressure regulation.

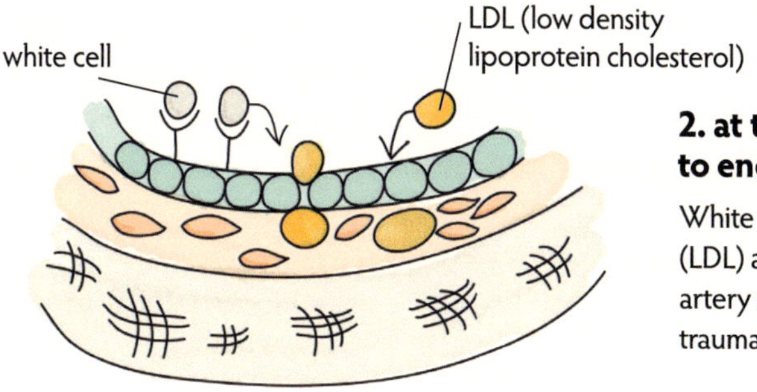

2. at the site of damage to endothelium

White cells and cholesterol (LDL) are drawn into the artery at the site of damage or trauma to the endothelium.

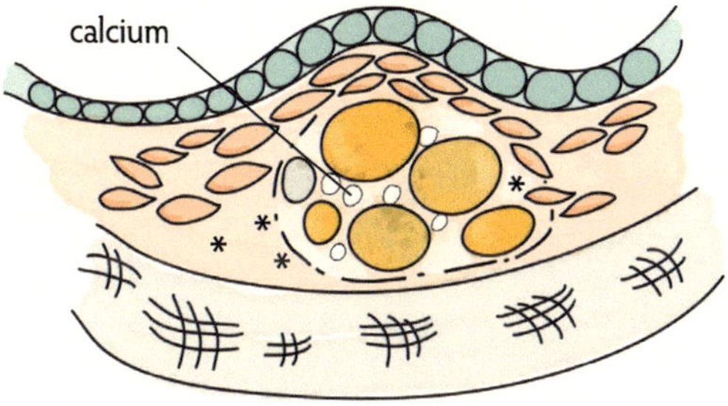

3. development of plaque

White cells and cholesterol collect in plaque as macrophages and lead to scarring. Calcium moves into scarred areas of plaque.

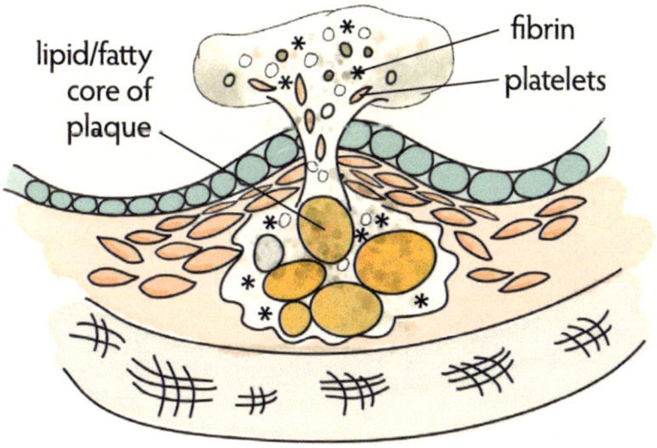

4. rupture of plaque and formation of clot (thrombosis)

Blood contents react with the contents of the plaque when it ruptures. A clot forms.

The **outer layer** is the main scaffold of the artery, and is made from **collagen**, the tissue that binds together almost all tissues in the body. The outer walls of the major arteries are, and need to be, very tough to deal with years of pulsating blood being forced through them. Interestingly, the stretch and recoil of the walls act as a secondary pump for the body, maintaining flow between heartbeats.

At a cellular level, minor damage to the inner lining of the artery leads to 'activation' of the endothelium. This means the endothelium presents proteins to the bloodstream, which can attract and hold white cells (leukocytes) which are the body's response to damage. The white cells are then drawn into the endothelial cells and from there, migrate into the space between the endothelial cells and the smooth muscle cells. At the same time, cholesterol is drawn into the wall of the artery, presumably as part of the healing process as cholesterol is needed for the construction of cell membranes. The leukocytes, which are part of the immune system, then mature to cells that digest foreign material. These mature cells are called macrophages and are the vacuum cleaners of the body.

The trouble is, the macrophages then start to clean up the low-density cholesterol that has also come through the area of 'activated' endothelium. These cells become full and 'stuffed' with fat and are now called foam cells, which age and eventually die, spilling their contents within the middle layer of the artery.

The spilt contents are components of the plaque along with free cholesterol and enzymes and cellular debris from the macrophages. The enzymes lead to micro-scarring, and with cellular debris contribute to a matrix, or scaffold, that can subsequently become calcified.

A collection of cholesterol, scar tissue and calcium forms within the wall of the artery. This is **atherosclerosis plaque**. Ironically, it starts as a process to heal the artery. Yet, in some cases, it progresses to causing problems, even death.

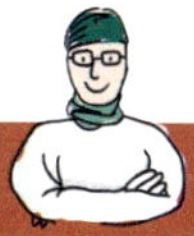

CASE STUDY – Prevention is better than cure

PENNY was 52 years old when she came to see me (WB). She was generally well and on no medication. She was a non-smoker and didn't have elevated blood pressure. She was concerned, however, because her family had a worrying history of premature coronary disease.

Her lipid profile was:

Total Cholesterol (TC)	6.1	ideally < (less than) 5.0 mmol/l
Triglycerides (TG)	0.6	ideally <2.0 mmol/l
High Density Lipoprotein (HDL)	2.1	ideally > (greater than) 1.0 mmol/l
TC to HDL ratio	2.1	ideally <4.0 ratio
Non HDL	4.0	ideally <4.0 mmol/l
Low Density Lipoprotein (LDL)	3.7	ideally <2.5 mmol/l

If we put these results into the Australian cardiovascular disease risk calculator, we see Penny's risk is estimated at one per cent in five years and she gets a green indicator.

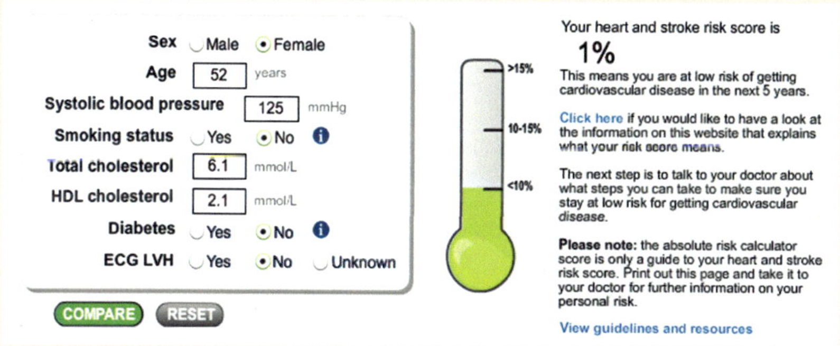

The important thing to remember here is that **a risk calculator doesn't predict the risk for an individual** patient. Rather, it provides the **rate** events occur in a **group of 100 individuals** with the same characteristics. This does not tell us **which** individuals will have the events.

Penny was well informed when she came to see me. She had already had a significant discussion with her general practitioner and had looked at my website to obtain information about scanning the heart.

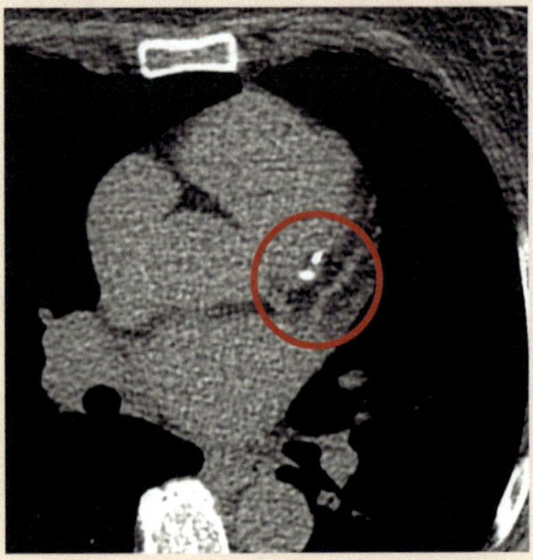

Her husband, who came with her, also decided to have his heart scanned. He was about the same age, with a similar lipid profile, had borderline high blood pressure and had a bit of weight on his tummy. He was the one who looked as if he might have the unhealthy arteries.

These were Penny's calcium score image (*above*) and results (*below*):

Scoring Results: Agatston Score Protocol				
	LAD	LCX	RCA	Total Coronaries
Score	71.45	30.64	141.35	243.44
#ROI's	2	2	14	18
AreaSq (sq.mm)	17.86	12.77	46.22	76.85

Her score of 243 is high for a young woman. For her age, the 90th percentile is 65! This result is three to four times higher, suggesting that Penny was probably the one out of 100, or the one per cent!

Although the results brought Penny to tears when she first heard this news, as the significance of having this knowledge sank in, she calmed down. There was no narrowing in the arteries and there had been no damage to the heart. And we had found what we had been looking for – to see if she had the same issues as others in her family. Although she did, **we had found the brake cylinder that was about to fail before the accident!**

We were able to institute therapy. For her, we were ahead of the game. There is little doubt that Penny found this process confronting but invaluable, and just to complete the story, her husband had zero calcium score!

ANSWERING YOUR QUESTIONS ?

what is a coronary calcium score?

Calcium scoring provides a sensitive indicator to the presence of atheroma (plaque, the fatty deposits) within a person's arteries.

It is an absolute number and there is a significant body of research that supports the premise that the greater the absolute coronary calcium score, then the greater the risk of an event that an individual carries.

Calcium is not the problem. Calcium is inert in arteries, so it can stay there. However, it is an indicator of a potential risk. The problem is the plaque build-up of which calcium is a component.

Over many years, work in demonstrating an association between the amount of calcium present in an individual's arteries and the risk of progressing to a major adverse coronary event means that calcium scoring has become a prominent and sensible marker in risk assessment – a very powerful negative predictive test (meaning the condition is not present).

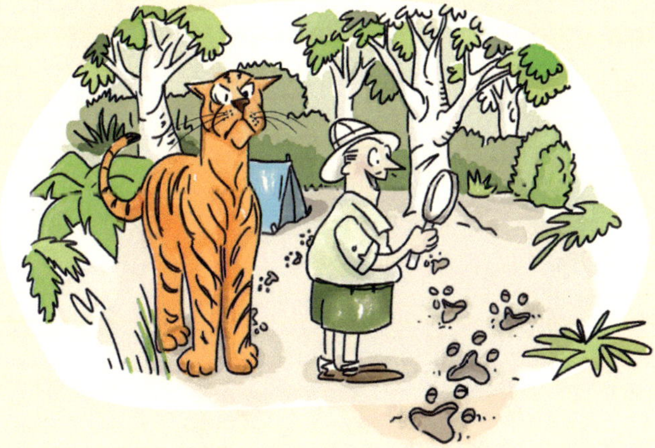

Calcium is simply the surrogate marker we use to give an indication of the process we are concerned about, the build-up of plaque within the coronary arteries.

I (WB) use the example that if, on pitching a tent in the jungle, we saw lots of tiger footprints, it would mean that tigers are around, and it might not be a great place to pitch the tent. Not seeing tiger footprints doesn't mean there are not tigers in the area but it certainly makes it a better place to pitch a tent!

Neither a normal stress test (running on a treadmill), nor a normal invasive coronary angiogram (when the contrast or die is injected directly down the arteries) can provide the same assurance, while "low cholesterol" "regular exercise", "good diet", "watching my weight" and "a healthy lifestyle" cannot come anywhere near to being as useful in predicting a low risk of an event as does a zero coronary calcium score.

In the 1980s, a new technology called electron beam computed tomography (EBCT) ignited renewed interest in evaluating the health of an individual's arteries. This so-called computed tomography (CT) has moved on a long way. Since about 2006, a new generation of CT machines has become available.

Today's CT scanners image the heart using a gantry system (a large ring) that spins x-ray heads and detectors around the patient at high-speed. Each rotation of image acquisition can obtain from 4cm to the full vertical distance of the heart. The speed of rotation is very fast – and continues to increase with improvements in technology. Because the heart is constantly moving, the faster the image can be acquired, the less blur and the better quality of the image. These new machines, with more detectors and faster rotation times, are being used with advanced technologies that reduce the radiation doses to below ordinary yearly background radiation.

A CT scanner is used to measure the amount of calcium (calcified plaque) in the coronary arteries. A zero score indicates there is none.

See page 295 for details

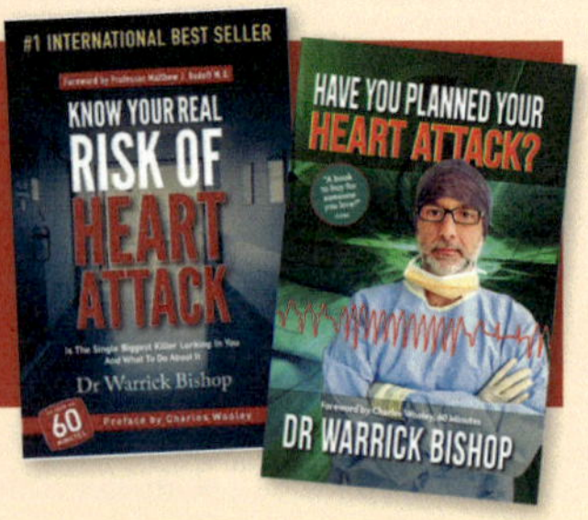

Don't let life get in the way of saving your life

Dr Bishop speaks with patient and fellow surfer, Brian

who turned 60 (mid-2020), is married with two young adult children. Born on Flinders Island, a small island in Bass Strait between Tasmania and mainland Australia, he has lived a physical, outdoors, manual-labouring life. The family story says that males in Brian's family do not live past 50 years of age on his father's side. Although his father died at 72, he had his first heart attack aged 49. This event damaged his father's heart and severely impacted the remainder of his father's life.

WB **The last couple of months probably have been confronting for you, Brian, and have led to you having a stent inserted into one of the arteries of your heart. A stent was placed in the beginning, or proximal part, of the left anterior descending artery. The left anterior descending artery is the one that runs down the front of the heart nearest the breastbone or the front of the chest wall. So, let's go back, Brian, and tell me the story about how all that came about.**

B *Over the years, when I was seeing my GP, he was generally very unhappy with my cholesterol results. And this went on for years and years. I didn't like taking the statins, but I did try on a regular basis and took them for quite a few years. Probably about three years ago, on a visit to my GP, I just asked him a question,* Was there anything available that actually looks at the arteries around the heart? *He said there was a thing called a calcium score. It all went over my head, but I thought,* That sounds interesting, *so I put it in my mind that I would get it done. But being a typical Aussie male, I just kept putting it off because life was getting in the way. Maybe thanks to the coronavirus, because we couldn't make our annual surf trip to southern New South Wales, I decided to get the coronary calcium score done. And basically, things unravelled from there. The calcium score came back. Not very promising. And then, pretty quickly, I was in to see you, and I was really glad about that.*

WB Well, from my side of the story, your GP, who's an excellent GP, made that arrangement for your CT scan. He then asked me to look in on it and offer some advice. Well, certainly, by looking at the scan, there was a suggestion that there could be narrowing in the arteries. Our test is not perfect for telling us about narrowings, but it does tell us if there's 'rust in the pipes'. And we got you in pretty quickly for a treadmill test. Do you remember that?

B *It was all very quick. And I'm pleased that it was.*

WB Well, we found surprisingly very little on your stress test. If you recall, you actually performed pretty well. I think this is an important reminder for people. If something doesn't feel right, it's probably worth getting it checked out. Tell me about the symptoms that you had as you ran along the beach, getting ready to go for a surf because we got a small replication of that on our treadmill test, and that was enough for us to go to the next step.

B *Well, I really had no chest pain, just a tiny little bit of breathlessness, but nothing that I thought was out of the ordinary. My main symptom was, when I was running up the beach for a surf, I could feel my heart getting substantially out of rhythm. I tended to ignore it because I had a history of ectopic heartbeats, and I just put it down to maybe that was worsening. As it turns out, it was different. So, pretty much, it was the heart substantially out of rhythm when I was running.*

WB So, in essence, really not a lot. When we put you through that treadmill test, you had a good exercise capacity, and there were not a lot of changes on the ECG. You did have a little bit of shortness of breath, but nothing staggering because you're pretty fit for your age. What we did see was a suggestion of some minor changes on the ECG, not a lot, but we also saw some of those extra beats that you were describing. And that was potentially lack of blood flow causing some irritability to the heart muscle. I said that we should have a look at your arteries in more detail. I think we did that within a week or so. Is that right?

B *I don't think it was even a week. It was very quick.*

WB We got you on some medication immediately to try to make you as safe as possible as soon as possible and we got you in for the invasive coronary angiogram where we squirted dye through the arteries. This procedure showed a very tight narrowing, about 95 to 99 per cent, in the artery running down the front of the heart. That particular location is referred to as the 'Widow Maker' because it has been the location of a ruptured plaque that's led to sudden, unexpected, cardiac death in blokes at a relatively young age. So, having found that narrowing, we kept you in hospital overnight. I organised for one of my colleagues who implants stents to open that artery the next day. Tell me how the angiogram was for you and then how you were emotionally that night and the next day.

B *Look, I found the whole process extremely easy. I was fairly relaxed through the whole thing. Even though they keep you awake, they give you a drug that makes you feel comfortable. There was no pain involved, and I found the whole thing really interesting. When you told me I needed a stent, I thought,* Good; we know what we're doing, *and I was rapt when you told me it would be done first thing in the morning because I thought,* Right, let's get it done, *and I wasn't going to be waiting around for weeks stressing about what might happen. So yeah, I really did find it quite easy, and the night in hospital, I loved it because I was getting full attention. It was really quite enjoyable, to be honest.*

WB Well, that's pleasing to hear from this side because we want to be caregivers who make the journey as smooth as possible. When I saw the narrowing in the artery, I could have thrown my hands in the air, saying, *Wow, that looks a bit scary; you could die.* However, as little anxiety as possible in that space is useful and assists in achieving the best outcome for everyone, so I suggested you stay in overnight to see what could be sorted out for you.

B *Yeah, I think that was a really good move. I cottoned on to it. Probably halfway through the night I thought that there might be a little bit more going on than what you had indicated. But, as I say, the whole process was really easy.*

WB Although you left getting a CT scan maybe three years longer than you should have, what I think is incredibly valuable from your story is that we can sort out these potentially life-threatening problems between nine to five, Monday to Friday, with clear heads, with clear thoughts, without ambulances, without that risk of heart attack and dropping dead because we had the chance to look at your arteries in advance of a problem occurring. I think that's an extraordinary opportunity, and your testimony shows just how valuable that is.

B *I look back at it now and think it was intuitive for me to go and ask because I had no idea if there was some way to look at the arteries – but there was something because of my family history, and also the doctor was never happy with my cholesterol levels. And so, to me, it just makes a lot of sense that if you can actually look at the arteries, why wouldn't you?*

WB One of the things that's really important to me if we find individuals who have problems with their arteries is to ask the question about other family members who could be at risk. So, do you have brothers or sisters who you need to speak with about getting checked out in a proactive way?

B *I have two sisters still alive. One of them has had a lot of major health issues unrelated to heart disease and is in quite a bad state. My sister in Adelaide, I did talk to her, because she reminds me of me a fair bit. And I mentioned to her that, you know, maybe she could think about asking about a calcium score. I'm not sure what she's thinking. The one big difference between her and me is her cholesterol levels have been substantially under control for years. So, I think at the moment, she feels pretty happy. But you know, from what I've learned, after reading your book, you just don't know. And if you can get a picture, it might tell you something you are totally unaware of.*

WB Brian, do you have any advice for others?

B *I'm an outdoors person; I'd always relied on physical strength to barge on through life. Having had this lesson, I'd say to people,* If you're a bit worried about it, and, you know, you're sort of noticing things that you're not quite sure, it might be worth talking to your doctor about having a calcium score done. *Certainly, I'm so glad that I did it because I think I was on the edge. So yeah, my advice is,* Don't tough it out so much and don't let the stresses of life and the busyness of life stop you from investigating. **It's really nice to know.**

WB Don't let life get in the way of saving your life!

B *Yeah.*

WB We will probably start surfing again in the next couple of weeks. I was out yesterday, and you have been given clearance to start surfing again.

B *Absolutely. And it was quite a bizarre feeling for me because I saw you on Friday and you gave me the all-clear, and that afternoon I was out in front of your house, on lovely little waves and just kept looking up at your home thinking,* Wow this is quite surreal. *I'd like to thank you very much for basically saving my life. That's the way I feel. So, thanks, Warrick; thanks very much.*

WB I was delighted to be involved, Brian.

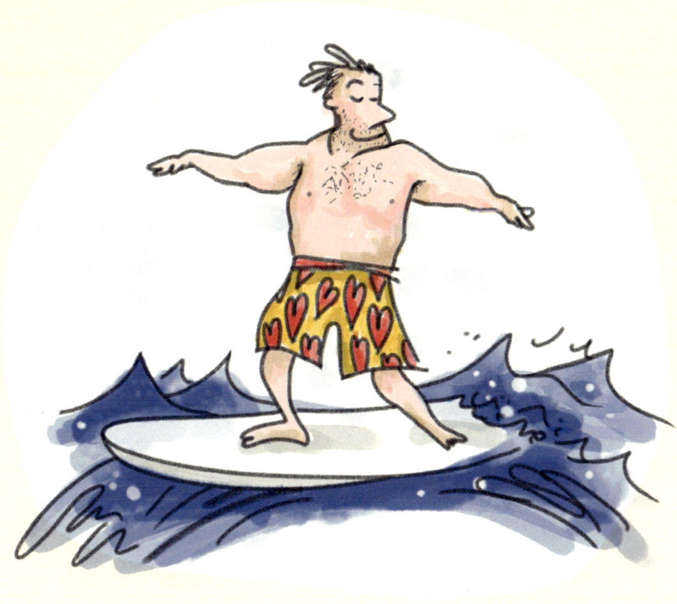

IMPORTANT POINTS

- Detection and treatment of coronary artery disease, historically, has been related to the presence of symptoms or the occurrence of a major coronary event.
- Plaque is the build-up of cholesterol and other matter within the arteries. This build-up can be patchy, tending to occur where there are points of stress, weakness and/or vulnerability in the artery.
- Plaque can be
  - flow-limiting, which generally, although not always, produces symptoms, or
  - non-flow-limiting, which will cause no symptoms.
- In either case, unstable plaque can rupture and a clot, which can block the artery, can form very quickly. When a seemingly fit and healthy person drops dead, during exercise, for example, it is often the case that the person has had an unstable non-flow-limiting plaque rupture – and therefore, no symptoms before the life ending event.
- Calcium has been observed in the arteries of living subjects for more than 80 years. While it is not the problem, it has become – through a test called a coronary calcium score – the standard marker for indicating plaque build-up within the coronary arteries.
- Technology has improved significantly in recent years and now dye/contrast can be injected during a CT scan to outline the coronary arteries in exquisite detail.

15 *CAD is the leading cause of death for Australians, responsible for taking a life every 30 minutes or on average 50 people per day. CAD is the second leading cause of death for Australian women – taking nearly more than three times the number of women than breast cancer and worldwide it is estimated that CAD is responsible for at least 1/3 of the deaths among women. see Heart Foundation: Coronary Artery Disease and Key Statistics: Coronary Heart Disease.*

16 *Libby P, Ridker PM, Hansson GK. Progress and challenges in translating the biology of a theory crisis. Nature 2011;473:317-25.*

17 *Preventative cardiology is a particular interest of Dr Bishop. In his first book, "Have You Planned Your Heart Attack?" (in the United States, "Know Your Real Risk of Heart Attack"), he argues for the increased use of cardiac imaging to see the health, or otherwise, of the coronary arteries before major cardiac events change, or end, people's lives.*

Time is of the essence in treating heart events, especially a heart attack.

chapter 5

THE CLOCK IS TICKING

A patient will present to a cardiologist in one of three ways,

- in the back of an ambulance, suffering chest pain from a suspected heart attack,

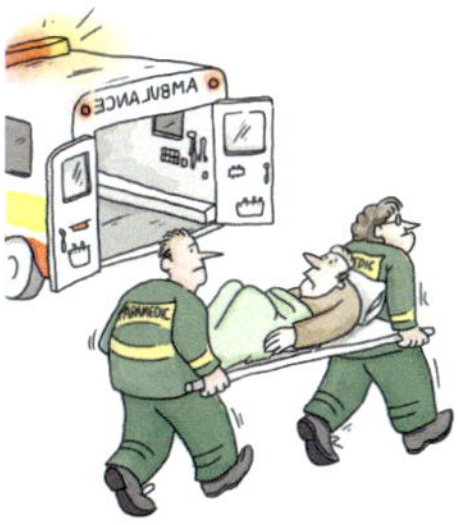

- in a more controlled way, in the cardiologist's consulting rooms after the patient has recognised a decrease in exercise capacity over time and then presents for evaluation, or
- in the most controlled way, by being proactive and having a heart scan ***before*** developing a symptom, thus allowing for appropriate management of any potential problem.

Whichever of the routes, the clock is ticking.

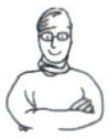

Before reading further, you might like to recall our earlier discussion on plaque, particularly pages 62-64.

heart attack

If someone

- has chest pain that is
  - central with a heavy and dull, or sometimes squeezing, quality
  - building up to severe, and
  - sometimes radiating down the arms,
- looks unwell,
- is suffering shortness of breath, and
- is sweating,

the person is having a heart attack and an ambulance should be called or the person taken to an emergency department, **immediately**.

Women may experience less typical indicators such as back, neck or jaw pain or tightness, shortness of breath and fatigue. Only half of the women who suffer a heart attack report chest pain.

Heart attack symptoms need to be recognised early and treated promptly and appropriately. However, individuals may not always exhibit 'typical' features. I (WB) have seen patients who have had pain in the left elbow, or pain between the shoulder blades, and even pain in their teeth as their 'version' of heart pain. Just be aware that if something is 'not right', it might be your heart and have it checked. (Please see Appendix 1 for further information on recognising the warning signs of a heart attack.)

The quicker the person arrives at an emergency centre, the quicker the condition can be diagnosed and treatment begun, and the more likely the person is to survive. Once an artery starts blocking then it's like a clock ticking. The longer the blockage 'ticks', the more heart muscle dies. Opening the artery to restore the blood flow saves lives. Time means muscle.

When a person presents suffering a heart attack, the culprit artery (or arteries) needs to be unblocked as soon as possible by using

medication	while most people live close enough to a centre with heart treatment expertise, a large number still live in the country. When time and distance constraints intervene, clot-busting drugs are used;
stent, a wire mesh scaffold	implanted in the catheterisation laboratory; often used when a single artery is involved.

After the patient has been stabilised

bypass surgery	often used when multiple arteries are involved, and the diseased area is relatively large. Rarely used at the time of the heart attack.

Fortunately, fewer people are presenting with heart attack symptoms because more people are in the second group, being checked at an early stage. This better scenario means cardiologists can manage a person's situation by trying to identify a problem before it develops. With appropriate recognition of risk factors and testing, many heart attacks are avoided.

scenario:

> *A 62-year-old man, who has reported to his GP that he's experiencing some chest tightness and shortness of breath when he climbs the stairs at work, is referred to his cardiologist.*

Dr Alistair:

> *Simply by the fact that he is a 62-year-old male who experiences exertional chest pain or tightness, it's highly likely that the symptom is due to his heart. One of the cardinal symptoms of heart disease is exertional chest pain or tightness.*
>
> *To evaluate this patient, I would take a* ***detailed medical history*** *to ensure that what sounds like a cardiac problem is not something else. I would also examine the patient for changes, such as in blood pressure or other abnormalities that would give an indication of an underlying cardiac problem.*
>
> *The patient would then undergo an* ***electrocardiogram*** *(ECG), an electrical tracing of the heart (sticky dots on the chest with wires that go to a computer to produce tracings of the heart's electrical activity). That tells me if there are any blockages or developing problems. The patient then would undergo some form of* ***effort testing****, such as an exercise test or an exercise stress ECG, with or without some imaging.*

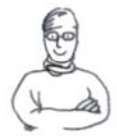

'Functional testing' tests the function of the heart. Continuing our car analogy, it is like taking the heart for a test drive.

This functional testing tries to reproduce the symptoms. Such testing indicates if there is a blocked or narrowed artery trying to supply blood to the heart.

Once this has been ascertained, I organise direct ***imaging*** *of the arteries using a dye (ink, or 'contrast') injected directly into the coronary arteries via access through the wrist or the groin using a catheter (a little plastic tube). As the dye passes through the arteries, a picture is taken that identifies exactly where an intervention is needed and gives information relevant to the kind of intervention.*

interventions

The most common procedure these days is the implantation of a **stent**. That would be in conjunction with the patient taking medicines; some, like aspirin, for the remainder-of-life, to ensure that the stent remains open.

While stenting is usually the preferred option and is far less invasive, the other is to perform the surgery, coronary artery bypass grafting, in which pieces of artery or vein from another part of the body are used to bypass the blockages.

Determining which procedure is used often depends on the number of blockages, where they are and their prognostic and functional significance. If the problem is in a main artery and there are numerous blockages – and particularly if the person is diabetic or has a loss of function of the heart muscle – bypass surgery tends to be favoured.

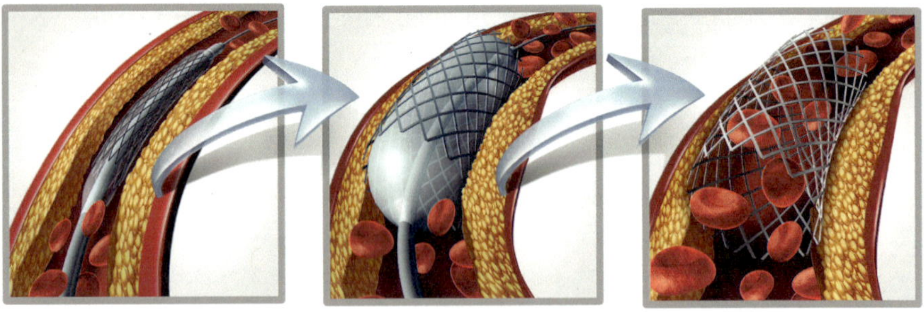

inserting a stent

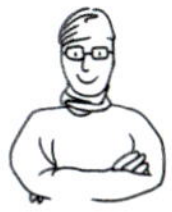

An adage, "if it isn't broken, then don't fix it", applies to hearts and our approach to deciding if we need to subject the patient to a procedure.

Two important trials, the Courage Trial[18] and the Ischaemia Trial[19], inform our management of patients who have stable symptoms. These trials tell us that for patients who have mild symptoms and less than about 15 per cent of their left ventricle (the main heart muscle) affected by poor blood flow, that optimal medical care – meaning aspirin, ideal blood pressure and cholesterol treatment – is as effective therapy as stenting.

Along the same lines, some good work[20] has shown how exercise can be as, or even more, effective than stenting in the right patient group. These trials really underline the importance of holistic treatment and care that involve the whole patient and not only the blocked artery.

ANSWERING YOUR QUESTIONS ?

what is a stent?

As we are discussing, a stent opens a narrowed artery to allow blood to flow freely. The stent is a fine metal scaffold that is inserted into a narrowing in an artery and then is expanded to keep the artery open.

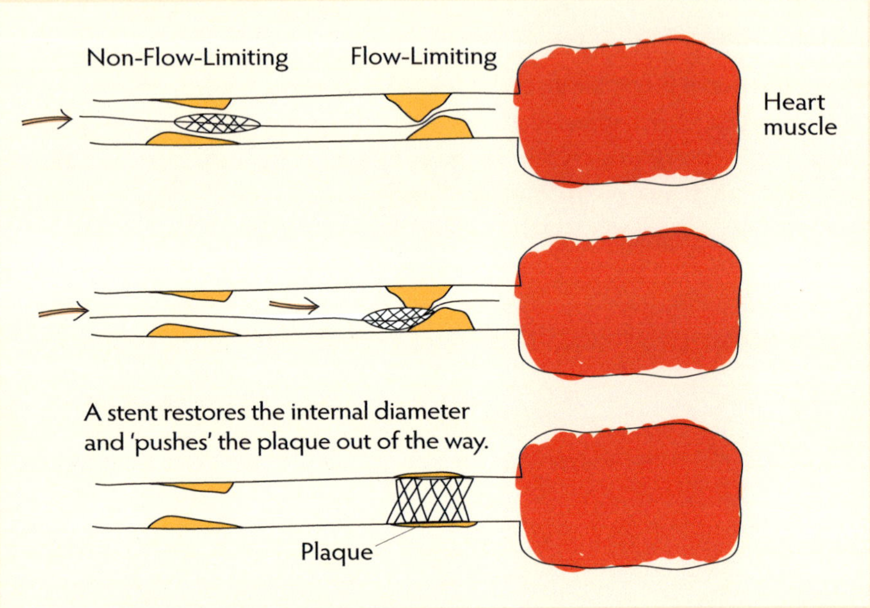

Stent implantation restores flow at the site of focal narrowing. However, it does not address non-flow-limiting plaque.

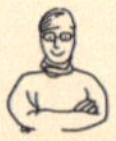

The implantation of a stent can be extremely effective at symptom management when there is a single isolated narrowing that has the characteristics to allow a stent to be inserted.
When we consider stenting in terms of prognostic management, the data are not quite so solid. A stent placed to unblock the narrowed portion of artery does not necessarily deal with the non-flow-limiting plaque that could be elsewhere in the coronary tree which may still subsequently progress and cause problems later.

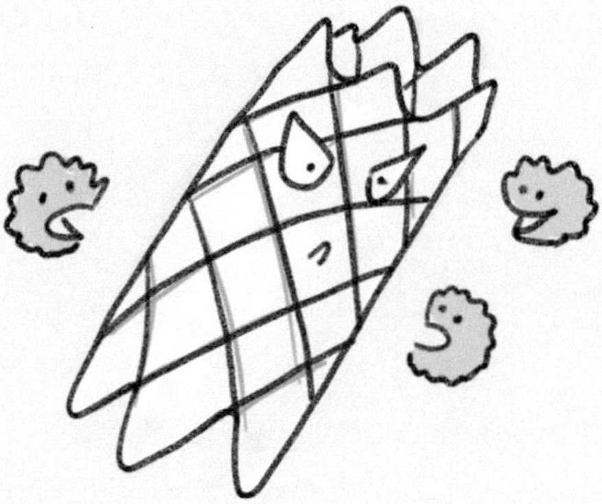

Although stenting is a terrific technology, there is a catch, and the catch is that the metal of the stent is seen as a foreign material by the blood's platelets. When platelets encounter foreign material, they interpret that as a cut in a blood vessel and go to work forming a clot to heal it. **Problem**! We don't want a clot in an artery as the clot will block it – again. **Bad news**!

In regular situations, the way to overcome the clotting is to give the patient drugs that prevent the platelets from clumping. Such drugs are called **antiplatelet** agents. Aspirin is the most well-known. However, and importantly, in the setting of stenting, two antiplatelet agents or **D**ual **A**nti **P**latelet **T**herapy (DAPT) are needed to prevent clot formation. Most often patients will remain on DAPT for a minimum of three months to a maximum of 12 months. During this time, as DAPT is preventing clot formation, the inner layer of the blood vessel grows over the metal struts of the stent, thus preventing the platelets from interacting with the metal.

This process starts immediately:

- by **one month** the process will have produced reasonable coverage,
- by **three months**, a pretty good coverage, and
- by **12 months** the stent, generally, will be completely covered.

What if the patient is already on an anticoagulant for, say, atrial fibrillation? Does the patient then take a blood thinner and two antiplatelet agents?

Think about the high risk of a bleeding complication that scenario may carry – medication to block the coagulation cascade **and** two medications blocking platelet function.

The objective is to minimise any risk of a clot forming in the stent while offsetting that against the risk of the patient having a problematic bleed. As the highest risk of stent thrombosis is in the first 30 days, patients will generally be on two antiplatelet agents as well as their regular anticoagulant during that time.

Depending on the complexity of the stent and other patient-specific issues, this triple therapy will be stopped after the first 30 days or continued for about three months when one antiplatelet will be stopped. One antiplatelet and the anticoagulant will be used until month 12. At 12 months, generally, the antiplatelet agent will be stopped, and the anticoagulant continued long-term.

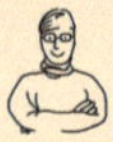

Remember, once your stent is in place, stay on your medications, and work with your cardiac rehabilitation team, your cardiologist, and your general practitioner to address traditional risk factors including considerations such as cholesterol, blood pressure and diabetes, as a means of looking after your stent, while it is looking after you.

A CLOSER LOOK

trials support the use of stents

Large, multicentre, randomised trials are more and more supporting the use of stents as much as possible. Very recently, the EXCEL trial[21] looked specifically at narrowing of the **left main coronary artery**, which is the biggest blood vessel that comes off the aorta to supply the left anterior descending artery and the circumflex artery. This single artery branches into two of the three main arteries of the heart.

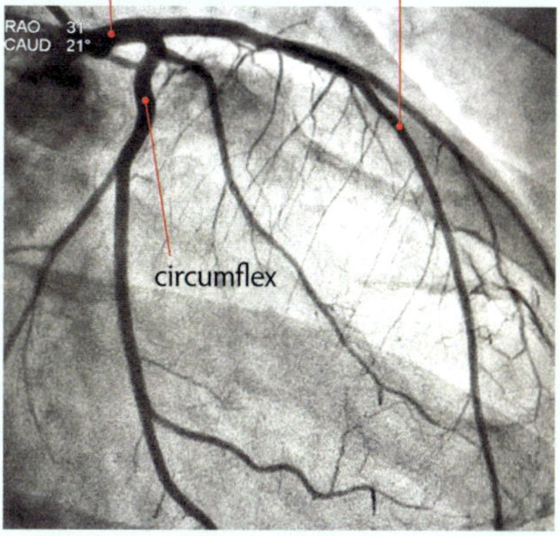

invasive coronary angiogram showing the left main coronary artery

Historically, left main disease meant surgery. The EXCEL trial followed several thousand patients over five years and randomised them to either stenting or bypass grafting. In the early stages (up to three years), the stenting group did better. Over the next couple of years, the bypass group did better, so that by the end of the study's five years of observation, results suggested that both strategies worked equally well. The observation is continuing now to 10 years.

Currently, when the cardiologist and the surgeon are deciding the most appropriate way to deal with the anatomy for a patient, either way is a reasonable approach. For certain patients, stenting in the left main now is a possibility. In the end, it will be a patient-specific decision based on the individual's specific clinical situation, clinical characteristics, and personal wishes.

Numerous new studies with refined parameters are being done as stent technology improves. The options are certainly becoming broader. Be in conversation with the cardiologist who implants your stent as he/she will be most up-to-date and, of course, will be familiar with your specific needs.

ANSWERING YOUR QUESTIONS ?

what is a coronary artery bypass graft?

A coronary bypass procedure (coronary artery bypass graft, CABG) uses an artery taken from the chest wall or the wrist, a vein taken from the leg, or sometimes both, to bypass a blockage in one or more of the coronary arteries (the arteries that supply the heart muscle with blood).

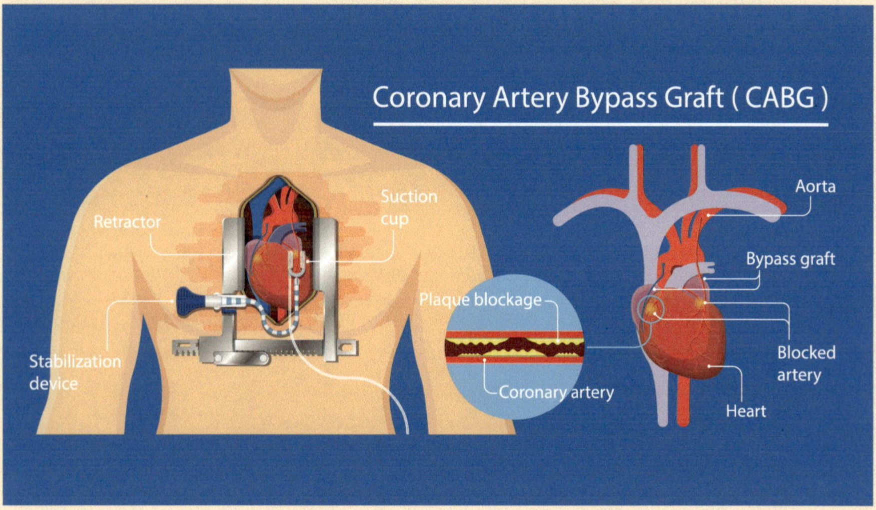

Chest wall arteries, particularly the left internal mammary artery (LIMA)[22], are the most used. The radial (arm) artery that supplies blood to the wrist is another common artery used while the most used vein graft is the saphenous vein taken from the thigh or calf.

The procedure, done under deep anaesthesia, usually takes between two and three hours depending on the number of grafts involved. Most bypass operations use a mid-line cut in the breastbone (median sternotomy), the ribs are pulled back with special retractors and the heart is placed on bypass using a special heart/lung bypass machine that oxygenates the blood and pumps the blood while the heart is rested during the surgery. Once the bypass has been performed, the heart is restarted, the circulation begins slowly, and the heart's natural pumping action is gradually restored. Throughout the operation, the patient is on a ventilator.

The patient spends one to two days in the ICU before being transferred to the ward. While in ICU, the patient's natural ventilation is restored. Pain and discomfort will be experienced post-operatively, in hospital and at home. Levels are variable and highly personal.

CABG is used for patients with ongoing angina, those not responding to medical treatment, or when stenting is not suitable for technical reasons. In most situations, it is performed to improve the person's chance of survival. Such situations include narrowing of the left main coronary artery, or where a significant narrowing occurs in all three coronary arteries, and with some damage to the muscle of the left ventricle.

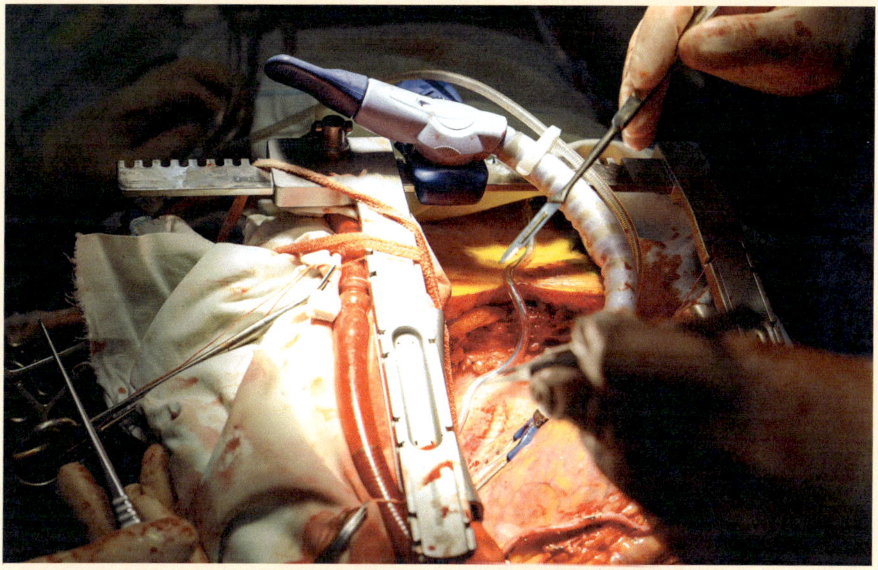

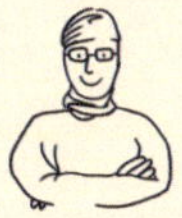

Although it remains a traumatic experience for the patient, bypass surgery is now an extremely efficient procedure that is becoming less invasive over time. However, a one to two per cent risk of dying from the procedure remains. A similar risk also exists for the person having a stroke or significant heart attack. Other complications include kidney failure, lung infections such as pneumonia, and blood clots in the lungs, or in the leg if a vein has been used. (For a patient's perspective, please see the Darren Lehmann interview, beginning on page 102 and re-read Ron's account beginning on page 15.)

IMPORTANT POINTS

- A patient will present to a cardiologist in one of three ways:
  - in the back of an ambulance, potentially suffering a heart attack;
  - in the cardiologist's consulting rooms, by referral, or
  - seeking to be proactive before even feeling unwell.
- Whichever way, the clock is ticking if the patient is suffering a blocked, or partially blocked, artery.
- If the person is suffering a heart attack, the artery or arteries need to be unblocked as soon as possible using
  - medication
  - implantation of a stent.
- The options for restoring the blood flow are stenting and bypass grafting. An ongoing drug regime is needed in both scenarios.
- Factors involved to determine how the blood flow will be restored include
  - the number of blockages
  - the position of the blockages
  - the likely prognostic outcome for the patient.
- If the person attends the cardiologist's consulting rooms, a detailed medical history is taken followed by
  - an electrocardiogram (ECG)
  - a stress test, and if indicated
  - imaging of the arteries

  to determine the name and extent of the problem.
- If the person is seen in a truly preventative situation, appropriate therapies can be started and any intervention can be planned for between 9 am and 5 pm, Monday to Friday. **Calm.**

18 *COURAGE trial - Boden WE, O'Rourke RA, Teo KK, et al. Optimal medical therapy with or without PCI for stable coronary disease. April 12, 2007 N Engl J Med 2007; 356: 1503–1516. DOI: 10.1056/NEJMoa070829*

19 *ISCHEMIA trial - The ISCHEMIA Trial, https://www.ischemiatrial.org/ (We are pleased to announce that the ISCHEMIA Trials have been recognized by the New England Journal of Medicine and by the Clinical Research Forum!) and*

Initial Invasive or Conservative Strategy for Stable Coronary Disease, David J. Maron, M.D., Judith S. Hochman, M.D., Harmony R. Reynolds, M.D., et al., for the ISCHEMIA Research Group April 9, 2020 N Engl J Med 2020; 382:1395-1407 DOI: 10.1056/NEJMoa1915922

20 *Percutaneous coronary angioplasty compared with exercise training in patients with stable coronary artery disease: A randomized trial. Hambrecht R, Walther C, Mobius-Winkler S, et al. Circulation 2004;109: 1371–1378.*

21 *Evaluation of XIENCE versus Coronary Artery Bypass Surgery for Effectiveness of Left Main Revascularization – EXCEL. Results were discussed at Transcatheter Cardiovascular Therapeutics 2019 (TCT 2019) the annual scientific symposium of the Cardiovascular Research Foundation. Another trial of interest is Five-Year Outcomes after PCI or CABG for Left Main Coronary Disease. November 7, 2019 N Engl J Med 2019; 381:1820-1830 DOI: 10.1056/NEJMoa1909406 (https://www.nejm.org/doi/full/10.1056/NEJMoa1909406)*

22 *also known as the internal thoracic artery (ITA)*

While cardiovascular risk factors do not automatically lead to cardiovascular disease, the more risk factors the person has, the more the likelihood problems will develop. Some risk factors cannot be modified but most can be altered to benefit the patient's health.

chapter 6

RISK FACTORS

The presence of cardiovascular risk factors does not mean a person will have, or develop, cardiovascular disease. However, the more risk factors present, the higher the likelihood of problems for that person. Coronary heart disease and stroke carry numerous risk factors[23] and many of them are shared. Some, such as family history, cannot be modified, while most can be improved with treatment and/or lifestyle changes.

non-modifiable risks

Common non-modifiable risks are family history, age, gender, and ethnicity:

- simply getting older is a risk factor;
- men have a greater risk of heart disease than women, but once passed the menopause, a woman's risk starts to approach a man's;
    - the outcomes worsen for women after menopause;
- people with African, Asian or Aboriginal and Torres Strait Islander ancestry are at higher risk than other racial groups.

As the risk of cardiovascular disease increases with age, risk associated with **family** and genes focuses on early onset in siblings and parents[24] rather than a 93-year-old great uncle. Early onset generally means having suffered CVD before the age of 55 for men and before the age of 60 for women. If both parents have suffered heart disease before the age of 55, a person's risk of developing heart disease can rise to 50 per cent compared to the general population. This is particularly so if there are other significant contributing issues such as a history of smoking or marked obesity.

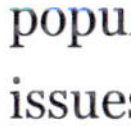

Alarm bells should ring, say, for a 48-year-old male whose older brothers all had stents by the age of 50. Such a history would warrant aggressive investigation and risk factor management to prevent what may otherwise be an inevitable event.

modifiable risks

Modifiable risks are those **acquired** throughout life. Common among these risks are

- smoking
- dietary decisions especially involving
  - fat, salt, and alcohol
  - low fruit and vegetable intake
- physical inactivity
- worsening cholesterol profile
- high blood pressure (hypertension)
- obesity
- diabetes
- mental issues and disadvantage.

According to Australia's Heart Foundation[25], most people do not associate these key risk factors with their heart health.

smoking

Smoking is one of the most significant risk factors and a major cause of heart disease, particularly for young people. Smoking – which includes passive smoking, vaping, using e-cigarettes, chewing tobacco, and using snuff:

- damages the lining of the blood vessels (the endothelium),
- can cause a stiffening of the blood vessels,
- increases fatty deposits in the arteries,
- contributes to atherosclerosis (narrowing and clogging of the arteries),
- increases the risk of clotting,
- affects cholesterol levels,
- promotes coronary artery spasm,
- accelerates the heart rate, and
- increases blood pressure.

None of these problems looks after the heart.

Smokers not only have more heart attacks, strokes, and angina than non-smokers, but also at a much younger age. A smoker is four times more likely to die of vascular disease (i.e., heart attack or stroke) and three times more likely to die from sudden cardiac death than a non-smoker[26]. Smoking kills 17 Australians every day through cardiovascular diseases such as heart attack and stroke[27]. Women who smoke are at a higher risk of heart attack than men who smoke.

Here's the kicker. If you quit, your risk of heart attack returns to the same as an age matched equivalent within two years. What a great deal!

dietary decisions

Australians of all ages generally do not eat enough of the five food groups and eat too much junk food which is high in salt, fat and sugar. Ninety-two per cent of Australian adults do not meet the recommended intake of vegetables (5+ servings of vegetables a day). Improving vegetable intake to meet the recommendation could reduce the risk of cardiovascular disease by 16 per cent.

physical inactivity

A sedentary lifestyle is associated with poor outcomes with respect to increased risk of coronary artery disease, as is being overweight and unfit. Four in every five (83 per cent) adults do not meet national physical activity guidelines, with females (84.2 per cent) being slightly more likely than males (81.2 per cent) to fail to meet these guidelines. While most people do not meet the physical activity guidelines, one in seven (14.5 per cent) do no form of physical activity. This proportion is rising over time.

worsening cholesterol profile

Although cholesterol is an essential building block of healthy cells, the risk of developing heart disease – heart attack, stroke, blocked blood vessels – rises and falls with the rise and fall of cholesterol levels in the blood. While cholesterol levels are mainly related to genetic factors, they are also clearly related to lifestyle factors, in particular consumption of saturated fats, lack of exercise and being overweight.

Three measurements are important in relation to the body's cholesterol levels:

- low density lipoprotein (LDL)
  - this is often called 'bad' cholesterol and it makes up most of the body's cholesterol. It can stick to the walls of arteries and cause the fatty build-up, plaque. Too much plaque leads to blockages of the arteries, preventing blood from flowing properly to the heart
- high density lipoprotein (HDL)
  - this is often called 'good' cholesterol because it carries LDL away from the arteries and back to the liver to be broken down and then passed from the body as waste
- triglycerides
  - triglycerides are the most common fat in the body. Along with increased LDL cholesterol or decreased HDL cholesterol, they can increase chances of the body developing fatty build-ups in the arteries, leading to a higher risk of heart attack or stroke.

More than two in five (41.9 per cent) Australian adults live with high cholesterol. The prevalence of high cholesterol peaks among those aged between 55 and 64 years of age.

high blood pressure

High blood pressure, or hypertension, is recognised as the leading risk factor for heart disease and/or the development of stroke and is also a common trigger for heart rhythm disturbances. A common problem in modern society, affecting about a third of adults[28], it tends to reflect a busy and stressful lifestyle. It can have a genetic predisposition that is made worse by unhealthy lifestyle choices. Almost 1.2 times as many males live with hypertension than females (36.2 per cent compared to 31.3 per cent). The prevalence of high blood pressure increases with age.

obesity

A person is classified as overweight if his/her body mass index (BMI) is 25 or over. Two of three (67 per cent) Australian adults are overweight or obese[29]. The prevalence of being overweight or obese is almost 25 per cent higher in males (74.5 per cent) than females (59.7 per cent) with these proportions increasing for both males and females over time.

Do not leave check-ups until you see your GP. Take out the tape measure and see for yourself. Waist measurements[30] should be no more than 94 cm for males and no more than 80 cm for females.

diabetes

Although diabetes can be hereditary, it also can be directly related to lifestyle choices. Diabetes occurs when a person's blood sugar level rises to a point where the pancreas, which produces insulin, is no longer able to keep the blood sugar in check.

People who have diabetes are two to four times more likely to develop cardiovascular disease (the leading cause of mortality for diabetics). Hypertension, abnormal blood lipids and obesity are significant contributing factors.

The potential for damaged nerves and blood vessels also opens the person to the possibility of a 'silent' heart attack, which lacks the typical chest pain.

Diabetes is a long-term disease and needs good control of dietary intake, particularly fats and sugars, as well as attention to proper exercise and weight control and, where indicated, medications.

mental issues and disadvantage

Stress can trigger heart attack or stroke and has been linked to high blood pressure, heart rhythm problems and diabetes.

Stress can

- push up blood pressure (increases the wear and tear on the arteries)
- increase cortisol levels (can increase sugar levels and push a person towards the diabetic spectrum)
- impact sleep (affects the body's metabolism, which affects how cortisol, sugars and lipids are activated within the body)
- cause people to comfort eat (generally not healthy choices), and
- cause people to drink more alcohol (can increase blood pressure, alter sleep patterns, increase the risk of developing atrial fibrillation).

In a major study, INTERHEART[31], psychosocial stress rate ranked third in importance behind serum lipids and smoking among the modifiable cardiovascular risk factors.

The impacts of socio-economic disadvantage and social isolation have been clearly linked to stress, mental health issues, anxiety and depression[32]. This becomes a 'double jeopardy' as the same individuals also have difficulties accessing quality food, education and medical care.

closing the loop

'Closing the loop' between rehabilitation and prevention is important and it extends to all the risk factors discussed in this chapter. For example, high cholesterol can run through families, as can behaviours such as smoking or poor eating. From a family perspective, it is important to mitigate these risks in other family members before they become full-blown problems.

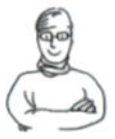

Blood pressure is a big consideration in relation to heart disease. Please shake up your family members to have it checked and monitored. High BP is directly linked to increased risk of heart attack, increased risk of stroke, development of cardiac failure, and development of atrial fibrillation – and do not forget renal failure. Without question, early detection and treatment prevent detrimental effects to the circulatory system over the long term and should be a health priority.

IMPORTANT POINTS

- The existence of cardiovascular risk factors does not mean the disease is present in the person or that it will develop. However, the more risk factors that are present, the higher the likelihood of problems.
- There are **non-modifiable** risks, including
  - family history
  - age
  - gender
  - ethnicity.
- There are **modifiable** risks, including
  - smoking
  - dietary decisions, especially involving
    - > fat, salt, and alcohol
    - > low fruit and vegetable intake
  - physical activity
  - high cholesterol
  - worsening cholesterol profile
  - obesity
  - stress, mental health, anxiety, depression
  - socio-economic disadvantage, social isolation.

23 the statistics and some of the information contained in this chapter are from the World Heart Federation website https://www.world-heart-federation.org/resources/risk-factors/

24 also referred to as first-degree relatives

25 Heart Foundation website, Key statistics: Risk factors for cardiovascular disease; https://www.heartfoundation.org.au/Activities-finding-or-opinion/key-statistics-risk-factors-for-heart-disease

26 Heart Foundation (Australia) website https://www.heartfoundation.org.au/Heart-health-education/Smoking-and-your-heart

27 Heart Research Institute: https://www.hri.org.au (health/learn/risk factors/smoking)

28 Heart Foundation: https://www.heartfoundation.org.au/Activities-finding-or-opinion/key-statistics-risk-factors-for-heart-disease

29 ibid.

30 Heart Foundation: https://www.heartfoundation.org.au/Heart-health-education/Waist-measurement

31 Effect of potentially modifiable risk factors associated with myocardial infarction in 52 countries (the INTERHEART study): case-control study. Prof Salim Yusuf, Steven Hawken, Stephanie Ôunpuu, Tony Dans, Alvaro Avezum, Fernando Lanas et al. published: The Lancet, September 11, 2004 (https://www.thelancet.com/journals/lancet/article/PIIS0140-6736(04)17018-9/fulltext)

32 Depression is a common illness worldwide, with an estimated 3.8 per cent of the population affected, including five per cent among adults and 5.7 per cent among adults older than 60 years. Approximately 280 million people in the world have depression. Depression is different from usual mood fluctuations and short-lived emotional responses to challenges in everyday life. Especially when recurrent and with moderate or severe intensity, depression may become a serious health condition. It can cause the affected person to suffer greatly and function poorly at work, at school and in the family. At its worst, depression can lead to suicide. World Health Organisation website: https://www.who.int/news-room/fact-sheets/detail/depression

There is no doubt that a significant cardiac event changes a person's life. However, there is a pathway of care available that can lead to a healthier and well-lived life.

THE CARDIAC REHABILITATION JOURNEY

YOUR WORLD HAS CHANGED

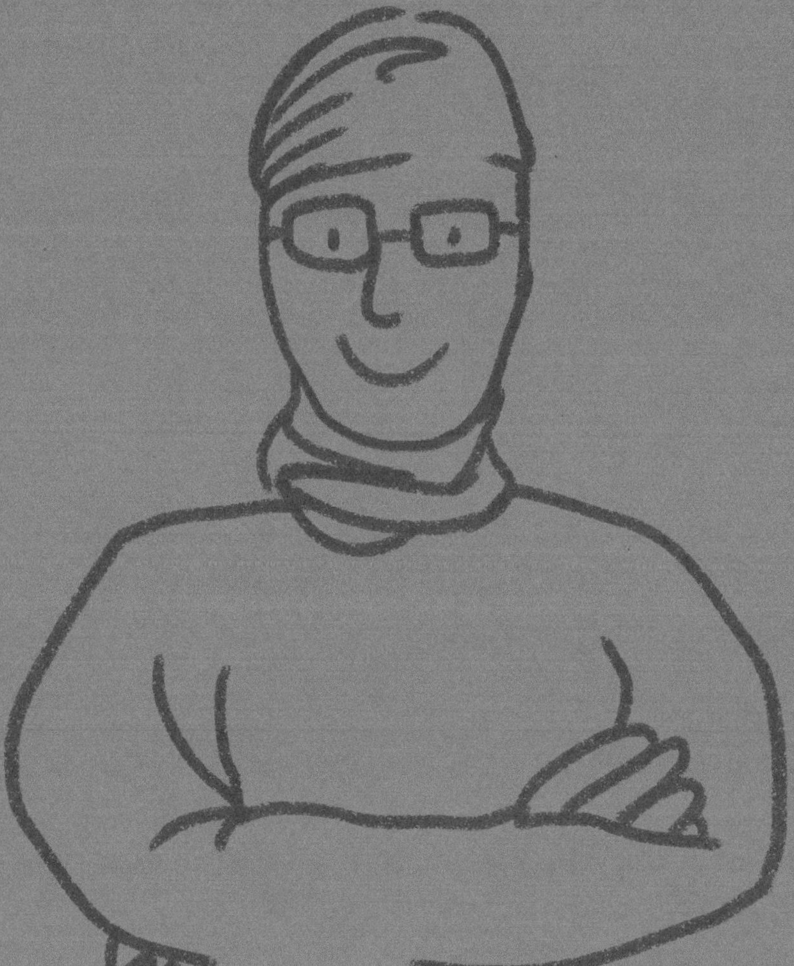

chapter 7

PATHWAY OF CARE

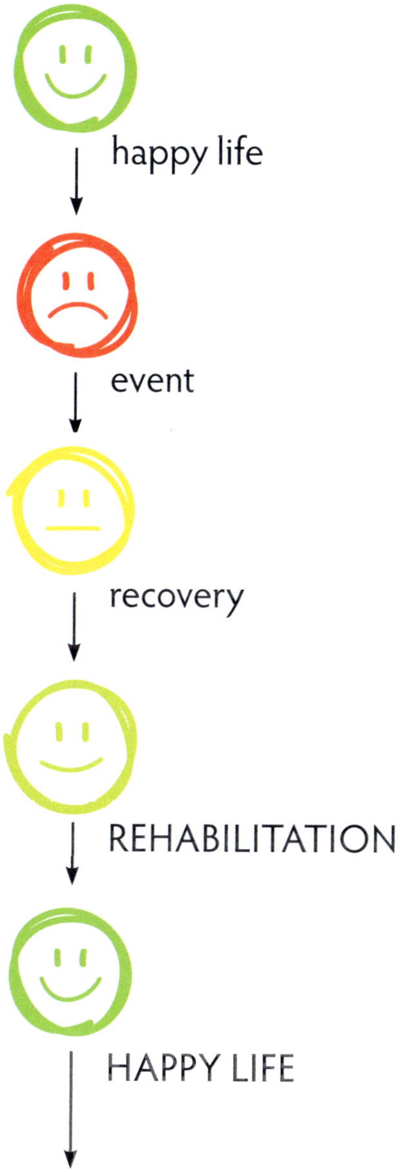

The greatest birthday present – a second chance

Dr Bishop speaks with Darren Lehmann[33]

a star in the annals of Australian cricket who was capped 27 times as a Test player (a free-scoring, top-order, left-hander). Darren also played 117 One Day Internationals, is a two-time World Cup winner, and, as a top-flight cricket coach saw his country to Ashes series wins in 2013-14 and 2017-18. He is married to Andrea and is the father of four[34].

In February 2020, Darren was anticipating an enjoyable, relaxing day for his 50th birthday watching his son, Jake, captain the Cricket Australia XI against the England Lions at Metricon Stadium, Gold Coast (Queensland, Australia).

He speaks about what happened instead, and the fundamental role of rehabilitation in making the most of his second chance at life.

D *I'm 50 years old, and on my 50th birthday, I had a heart attack.*

I played cricket all my life – 30-odd years I've been involved in cricket. I played for 20 and then have been coaching for the past 10 years with various teams. So, cricket has been my life, but all of a sudden, things change, you know. February 5 (2020), 4:30 in the morning I woke up with cold sweats and something's really heavy on my chest.

Oh God!

And I don't mind telling people that I always was a smoker and quite a heavy smoker. And I thought, Well, I'll go have a cigarette and see if it makes it feel any better.

And I didn't have the cigarette, and I went: Wow, if I don't want a cigarette, I must be in some sort of trouble.

So, I rang the doctor[35] and they got the ambulance straight around. And they gave me a spray called GTN (glyceryl trinitrate[36]) – I always call it GnT (gin and tonic), but it's GTN, as you well know.

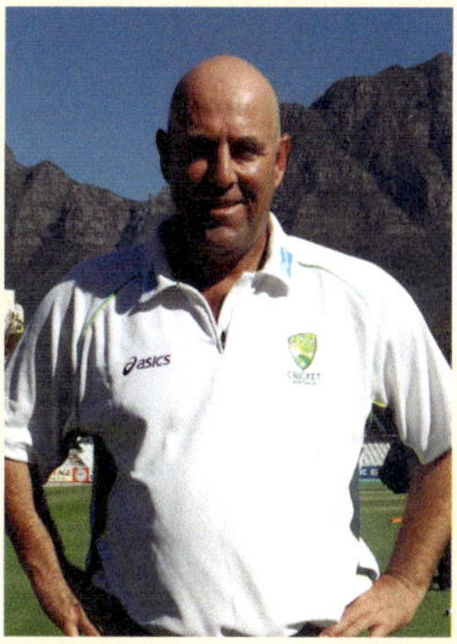

They gave me a spray first time and it sort of eased off a little bit of the pain, and especially the chest pain. And they waited five minutes and gave me another. The paramedics were fantastic, talking me through what was happening. And then they gave me a third spray and I felt really good. And I said, Thanks very much, lads, off you go. Don't worry.

And they said, No, no. You're coming with us. You're in a bad way. *And I went,* Well I feel good. What's wrong? I'm a 50-year-old. I can't be having a heart attack. This is ridiculous.

Anyway, I agreed to going with the 'ambos' and you know, an hour later I was in Gold Coast public hospital[37]*, and getting an angiogram done. And then, all of a sudden, the tests come back, and they say,* You've had a heart attack, and you've got blockages in three arteries. We're going to actually open you up and you're gonna have triple bypass surgery. *The operation was the next day – and a week later I was home.*

It was just a surreal experience, not really understanding but trusting what the doctors were saying. I'm just so thankful that I did.

Darren explained to Dr Bishop that looking back there might have been a warning sign or two. Before the heart attack, he would have a 30-40-minute nap after training or other physical activities.

D *I walk or bike every day, and I still do that now, but now I can breathe. It's just amazing that you don't know. And then you get these new arteries in your heart, and you can breathe again. That was the big change.*

If shortness of breath worsens or your exercise capacity diminishes, gradually, it's like when your kids grow up. As you see them every day, you don't notice how quickly they are growing. It's the uncles and aunties who recognise the difference. So, symptoms such as reduced exercise capacity can creep up.

WB It sounds like it crept up on you.

D *We live in quite a hilly suburb in Brisbane. I'd go walking and by the end of it I was really short of breath. Tired and, you know, couldn't keep going. But now it's fantastic. I go up these hills, and yeah, my heart rate gets up there, but I'm up and down and I keep going. I stop when I want to stop now, not because I have to stop.*

You know, I had what they call the widows, widows ...

WB Maker. Widow's maker.

D *That's right. Thank you. And that's another thing I have noticed since the operation, I forget a lot of things now. I find it hard to pick out words or remember things. They're starting to come back and they said that's just one of the by-products of open-heart surgery.*

This (the widow's maker) is what you see on TV – the reports of someone dropping dead on the footy field, or a lady riding a bike, suddenly having a massive heart attack and they can be as fit as anything. Heredity is a cause, and obviously, lifestyle. My lifestyle wasn't great, and I take full responsibility for that. I've had to change that. Even so, heredity is one of the biggest things.

After diagnosis, Darren was moved to The Prince Charles Hospital[38] in Brisbane and operated on within a couple of days by cardio-thoracic surgeon Dr Peter Tesar and his open-heart surgery team. Dr Bishop asked about the experience.

D *You don't cruise through it. You have a lot of questions because you don't understand, although they explained it well to me. The scary bit was probably the kids and my wife, you know. That day we were supposed to catch up for a great birthday party dinner. And that changed in the morning. All of a sudden, we are meeting in a hospital.*

Darren said the medicos had a calming influence on him because they explained what was happening so well. The pain came from having his chest sawn open. The hardest part, though, was the mental aspect.

D *The mental side of it was the tough process. My family members were great support. You know, you're scared because you could leave them behind. You're going into open-heart surgery, but what if it goes wrong? You just don't know, do you? Having said that, the doctors and nurses and all the staff were fantastic.*

Darren stayed in hospital a few days longer than the normal 5-7 days after by-pass surgery. Due to his history of smoking, the doctors wanted to ensure that he was breathing properly. His healing has taken time.

D *It was a long process. I mean, I only feel good, really good, now, in terms of physically. I still have the mental scars, but the side you notice is making sure the physical scars are healed and there's no infection.*

Basically, I spent 12 weeks just rehabilitating. ***I was so lucky to have a rehabilitation course at the hospital, running out of St Vincent's Hospital***[39]***.***

It goes through all you need you know, such as

- *dietary requirements,*
- *coming to understand the pills you're on – I've got so many pills now I don't know what all of them are but I know they do something for me,*
- *changing the way you think, your lifestyle,*
- *psychology,*
- *the physio, twice a week.*

It was a great course. You do it for six weeks. I recommend anyone do it if you get a chance, *mainly because I got to speak to people suffering the same issues as me. There were a couple of people younger than me, but most of them were, you know, I would say, 70 plus. Discussing how they were feeling and having open dialogue with other people and patients about what you have been through was very therapeutic for me.*

WB It sounds as if rehab was a very supportive, educational process for you. In relation to your smoking, did rehab require you to quit or did you make the decision yourself?

D *No, it was pretty easy – when you're sitting there with an open heart and coughing up crap. That was an easy one.*

The rehab came about because they offer the service and recommend people do it. They don't say you have to do it. ***Because I was in the unknown, and how I was feeling mentally, as well, I wanted to get a better understanding of the whole issue and especially the heart.***

For me, it was a great educational process.

You had twice a week, Tuesdays and Thursdays.

You do an hour of physiotherapy involving walking and numerous exercises to get you moving again.

And then you have an hour and a half lecture. That might be about the heart, or the drugs you are taking, or the operation itself, or it might be on nutrition.

On the mental side of it, the family side, you can have your partner come in as well. I almost think that should be compulsory, not recommended. There you go. That's how important it was for me to get through those issues.

I think rehab is a must-do for everyone. *I think you have to do it. Part of the discharge thing should be to sign-up for the rehabilitation part.* ***It was so good for me to understand what I'm feeling and why I'm feeling it and for the conversations with fellow open-heart surgery patients.***

WB Your overall experience sounds like a mixed blessing, like an extraordinary event that has changed the way you view things in a positive way.

D *Yeah, that's totally correct. I wouldn't wish a heart attack on anyone, but for me, it's a second chance of life and enjoying what I've got – not what I want to try and achieve, what I've got – and really simplifying that.*

I've got to a stage where I'm still coaching a cricket team but if that went tomorrow, I'm not too worried. I'm trying to learn how to fish. The only problem with that is I've got all these hook-marks in my fingers. ... I'm learning stuff I've not done before. I like that. It's really stimulating. And I'm seeing another side to life.

So, I think it was a blessing in disguise. While I don't wish it upon anyone, you just get a chance to re-evaluate your life, where you're going and to only keep the people who are important to you.

Charity work has always been a big thing for me so I'm throwing myself more into that as well. Because I'm fortunate enough to have a second chance, you want people to have as much as you possibly can.

WB It's an extraordinary sequence of events. One of the things that you mentioned are the good days and bad days, and I hope, and I get the sense, that you're probably having more good days than bad days now. My experience is that I think that some of those feelings people describe are part of a grieving process. We grieve an awareness of loss of health; we grieve we are not immortal. And grieving is a normal thing with loss. While we don't put a term to it normally, do you think grieving is part of the process you went through?

D *Looking back now, and the way you put it then, that is probably correct.*

For me, it was a case of going, Wow! How many people am I'm going to hurt through this? *and realising all you've got to concentrate on is yourself getting better, and you'll feel better. Then you can actually help people again.*

You can't look back. And as you said, I do have my bad days. Less and less. You know, bad days. It might be once a fortnight now. That's getting less. It was once a week, going back a few months.

Everyone's talking about COVID, and I know it's been a world-changing event, yet open-heart surgeries are like COVID in that you are isolated, basically for three months. You don't drive; you don't do anything. You are just recovering, slowly getting back into day-to-day living. So, it certainly is a wake-up call.

But with the grieving process, ***you are probably leaving one life behind and starting another one****. And that's probably the best way to put it really. It's hard to put in words, isn't it? Everyone* *says, with grieving, someone's died. Well, in essence, you sort of have because they've given you a new set of tools, a new engine, to start again and have a second crack at it.*

WB Some practical things, now. How are you going with your tablets? Any side-effects? Any problems?

D *No, I've been lucky with all my tablets – blood pressure tablets, warfarin. I go to the cardiologist again this week. Hopefully, I will be off warfarin, which means a stop to all those needles*[40] *every week, and back on Xarelto*[41]*, which I have been on before with my deep vein thrombosis (DVT). I know that it's a better tablet, although obviously, you don't get hit in the head while taking Xarelto*[42]*. I'll get back to that which will lessen the number of tablets. One tablet instead of a five-and-a-three or a three-and-a-three-and-a-one-half. I'm going to be on a lot of them for the rest of my life. That's okay; I understand that.*

I've got tablets in the little pill boxes. I think this is important, to remember which day you're at because some of the things with my memory is I forget what day I'm at.

I've got a little two-week travel box, which is quite small, which I reckon is very important. I keep that with me all the time. And I've got the one in the bathroom, which carries a month. So, I've always got six weeks of medications. I always like to have that much just in case something happens, or I've got to go somewhere. My job involved quite a lot of travel. I don't travel as much anymore. I haven't been out of Queensland since Australia Day this year[43]*. So, I've been a little bit lucky there, but that's because of COVID, and everyone's in the same boat.*

WB And, what about life at home? And how's the family now living around you? How are your relationships?

D *Relationships are stronger than ever. Because you almost lose something, relationships are stronger than ever. That's been a really interesting one. Then, having to deal with some of the issues that come up post heart attack. For probably three months, even though* *you know you get a second chance, the concentration span is not there. Things that frustrate me, I just say it, and I don't think about it sometimes. And then I go,* Well, I shouldn't have said that, like that. *You, and others, need to understand that that's just part of the rehabilitation, I suppose. And now, I can concentrate a lot more. But I wouldn't say I can concentrate for hours on end. You know, if I'm in a conversation like this, you've probably got me for 30 minutes in all. So, the family members know, and they sort of see it in me. When I might be a little bit frustrated, they give me my space and they'll say,* Go for a walk, Dad *or* Take the dog for a walk *or something. The cues come from them. They've been unbelievably supportive.*

WB As we come towards the end of our time together, are there any particular points from your own journey that you would like people to think about?

D ***The five days, post-operation, are some of the hardest days you'll go through. Physically, that's the toughest time.*** *And I can't commend the nurses or the doctors enough, putting up with me for those days. You're on drugs and different pain killers; you're constipated, you know, for a while, then you're not. They're dealing with those things all the time.*

They know each day's going to get better because they've seen it with so many patients, but you say, No, it's not; it's not getting better, *but gradually it does. The little increments over that period are quite important.*

Once you get home, rest*; it is an important part of the recovery process.*

Then, take yourself out for that hour a day. I think, starting, I could only walk 250 metres and then 500 m. Then it went to a 'k'[44]*, then 20 minutes and then half hour, then 40 minutes and then an hour. Don't try to push it too much. When I did my first walk, it was to the shops, about 250m away. And I thought,* Yeah, I'll walk home. *So, that was say 500m but I was only supposed to 250. I got home and I was just so out of breath. I'm like,* Oh, this is not good.

I'd say be patient with it.

If I had one bit of advice, apart from the rest – and make sure you listen to everything – it would be do the rehabilitation course. That'd be number one.

Yep. All the pain and the understandings.

The most important one for me was understanding –

- ***the operation,***
- ***the drugs you're on,***
- ***why you're on them,***
- ***what happened,***
- ***the heart and how it works,***
- ***the conversations you have in that course.***

Again, I would say it should be compulsory, whether you have a stent or open-heart surgery.

WB Well, the research supports that. So many people echo your sentiment, and it is an incredibly important component of the overall care.

Is there anyone you'd like to thank, particularly? You have said the ambos were fantastic. You said the docs were good. And you said the nurses put up with you, the physios flogged you and the rehab was great. Is there anyone in particular you want to thank?

D *The one person is my wife, Andrea. She's a nurse by trade, so she was quite calming especially when I was having bad thoughts of* Why is this happening? *or* Why is that scar not healing? *There were a couple spots on my arm that were red and inflamed and I had to go on antibiotics.*

Others include the local GP for reassuring me. All the people who had me day-to-day. The specialists were fantastic, and I can't speak highly enough about all the doctors and nurses.

But, you know, in the general day-to-day feeling of ups and downs, my wife and children for giving me the space to heal, both physically and mentally. You need that, you definitely need that. Nothing's too uptight or worrying now, but we're six months down the track. So, it does take a while. And, as I said, I'm still going through that process because there are days where I don't feel mentally quite right. As the doctors and everyone have said that it will take a year, maybe a year and a half, to be feeling really good about everything.

WB When we spoke about getting together for this interview, I did invite Andrea to join us. So, even though she's not here, what do you think would be her headline from this process?

D *It's time to slow down. Look after yourself and not others. And that's probably where you have the wake-up call. I was always worried about everyone else and probably not looking after my own health well enough. That would be the one thing she would probably say, and spending time with people who really mean a lot rather than other people who allow you to get to where you want to get to from a work position.*

So, really understand that life and families are a lot more important than jobs. We've all got to have jobs, I know, don't get me wrong, but just understand that the reason we are on this earth is to have a great family and enjoy what's a beautiful country and beautiful world.

WB Well, that sums up everything. I invite you to say goodbye.

D *Thanks for having me, Doc. Hopefully this has given you a little insight into what's transpired in my life over the last six months.* ***To everyone who goes through what I've been through, good luck. It does get a little bit easier each day. Just listen to the doctors and the nurses.***

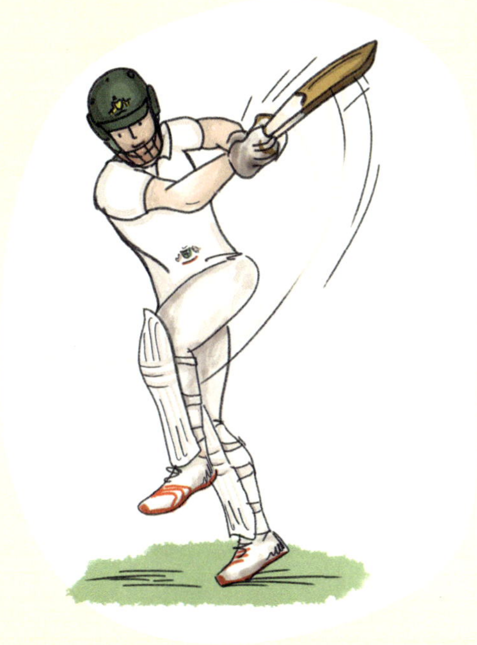

IMPORTANT POINTS

- Be aware of warning signs.
- Coronary artery bypass graft surgery, a painful and bewildering experience, is made bearable by the expertise, support and calm assurance of the highly trained and experienced medical team.
- **A rehabilitation program is essential to immediate and on-going recovery.**
- Ask questions. Take the advice given.
- Give yourself time to allow the recovery process to unfold.
- Be grateful for being given a second chance at life and for those who support you on the journey.

---

33 *This is an edited portion of the interview. Another segment features later in the book.*

34 *In 2020, a 28-year-old son lives in South Australia, a 25-year-old daughter is in Melbourne, Victoria, and 18-year-old twins live at home in Brisbane, Queensland.*

35 *Darren was staying at a hotel on Queensland's Gold Coast at the time.*

36 *used to treat chest pain (angina)*

37 *Gold Coast University Hospital, Southport*

38 *The Prince Charles Hospital is a major teaching hospital on Brisbane's northside with a specialty in cardiac and respiratory medicine and cardiothoracic surgery.*

39 *St Vincent's Private Hospital, Kangaroo Point, Brisbane*

40 *blood was taken every week to check the thinness of Darren's blood – international normalised ratio (INR) is a worldwide standardised test for measuring a person's blood clotting speed to reflect warfarin levels.*

41 *the blood thinner, rivaroxaban, a one-pill-a-day drug, which does not require blood test monitoring*

42 *as this is a blood thinner, the patient does not want to sustain an injury that bleeds*

43 *seven months at the time of the interview*

44 *one kilometre*

Change or chance? The decision is yours!

chapter 8

ARE YOU PREPARED TO CHANGE?

An honest answer to this important question – *Are you prepared to change?* – is the beginning of taking care of yourself, of effective rehabilitation and recovery, and long-term improved health. In almost all cases of significant heart disease or event, modifiable risk factors have helped bring you to your current state of health. The way forward is a forked road:

- do you live with your high-risk factors which are likely to worsen the disease or repeat the event, or
- do you embrace rehabilitation as the beginning of new habits for a better quality of life?

This improved quality of life goes well beyond taking drugs, as helpful as they are, for the remainder of your life.

While there is no question that prevention is better than cure when it comes to heart attack or any other heart problem, significant change is not always easy and, unfortunately for many, the 'best will in the world' needs some help.

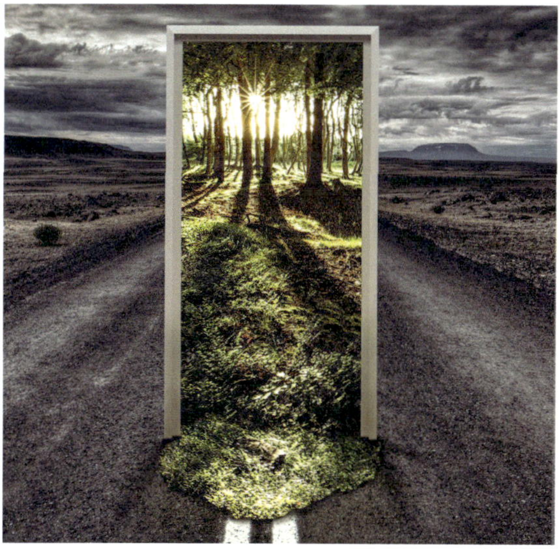

The good news is, there is plenty of help available. Importantly, such assistance can start in the cardiac rehab program where:

- support is available from the medical staff, and the journey is shared with other participants and the family who engages with the program;
- identification of mitigating social circumstances can be explored and supported by social worker input;
- financial pressures that may impact ability to eat well, engage in exercise or even afford medications can be identified and addressed, and
- identification, intervention, support, and monitoring of low mood or depression can receive attention.

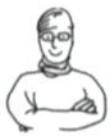

There can be multiple barriers to change. The more open you are in helping to identify those barriers the greater the opportunity is for help to be forthcoming. <u>So, please, speak up.</u>

change is possible

We have already discussed modifiable risk factors. Let us now turn our attention to how these old habits can be changed, and their benefits. For all modifiable behaviours, education is the best place to start.

smoking

Quitting any method of smoking is not an easy thing to do. Few people can go 'cold turkey'; for most people it requires planning, persistence and patience.

Advice from the cardiologist and general practitioner can be very effective in modifying smoking behaviours. General practitioners are important here as they see patients more frequently than the cardiologist and can coach the patient. Programs such as QuitLine[45] can also provide terrific advice and encouragement.

Dr Alistair:

I try to engage with the patient at the outset, asking if the person recognises that smoking has contributed to his or her current state of health.

I ask if the person is genuinely open to change. If the answer is "yes", I follow through with good information and I strongly support the person throughout the change.

If the answer is "no", I don't push too hard as I don't want to alienate the patient who I might be able to help with other modifiable risk factors. I hope that eventually the person will be prepared to take some action in relation to quitting.

As the starting point for this conversation is my good relationship with the patient, it can happen at any time. I would prefer it earlier rather than later. However, it's better later than not at all, if it is going to threaten our relationship and other health benefits.

Although smoking causes serious damage, over time, stopping smoking effectively reduces cardiovascular risk to close to that of a person who has not smoked[46]. Quitting smoking has the added advantage of saving money, as in most parts of the world it is a very expensive habit, and it also protects the health of you family, friends and colleagues.

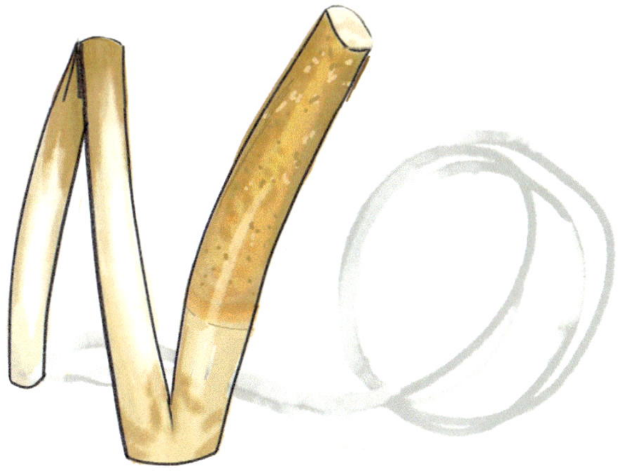

physical inactivity

The Heart Foundation (Australia)[47] recommends an accumulation of a minimum of 30 minutes a day, on most, preferably all, days of the week, exercising to a point of moderate intensity (heart rate rises but not to a point of breathlessness) for people 65 years and older. Balance and flexibility exercises should be incorporated most days and specific strength exercises should be done on two-to-three days of the week. And don't sit for too long.

Regular exercise is as effective as an antidepressant medication for mood[48]. And, so begins a list of significant benefits that not only assist heart health by reducing the risk of heart disease and heart attacks, but also incorporates preventing and managing a range of conditions and diseases that include some cancers and Type 2 diabetes as well as depression.

Exercising regularly, to a level with which the patient is comfortable, is the most important consideration and the best starting point. Exercise that is either too intense or not intense enough results in reduced health benefits. Another crucial factor is that exercise is not a short-term proposition; it needs to become a part of daily life.

Encouragingly, 'exercise' includes everyday movements such as walking to the shops or taking the stairs as well as more organised activities including sports, walking groups, yoga or attending a gym. Maybe even more importantly, it includes activities that a person already enjoys. And the other good news is that anyone can increase physical activity at any age and from any level of fitness.

Please just don't miss the chance to be active.

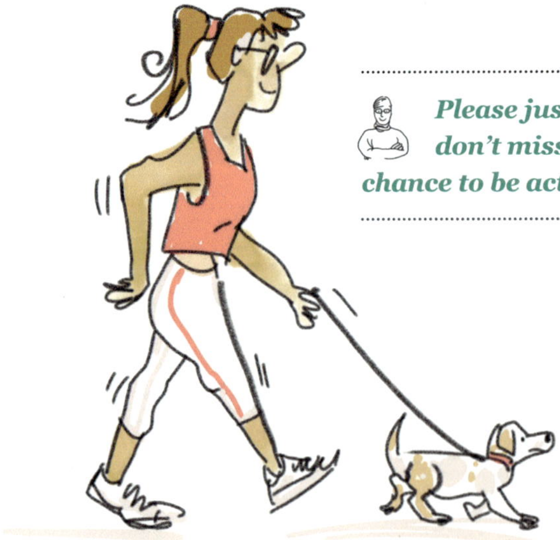

Sedentary behaviour is a big problem. Evidence says that many CVD patients engage in high levels of sedentary behaviour[49]. Additionally, it has been shown that among CVD patients, those who lead a more sedentary lifestyle are at increased risk of premature mortality (death)[50].

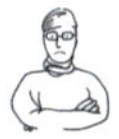

For CVD patients, who are already at increased risk, sedentary behaviours are particularly concerning.

Many patients, and especially those with diabetes, benefit from the advice and support of an exercise physiologist who can manage their exercise program in a structured way. *(also, please refer to chapter 13)*

worsening cholesterol profile

The body cannot live without cholesterol as it is a building block of the walls of the cells within the body and is also important in the production of hormones. Produced in the liver, it is water insoluble and floats in the body. Lipoproteins carry cholesterol to the tissues and back from the tissues to the liver. While most cholesterol is formed naturally within the body, it is also in the foods we eat.

The three ways of lowering cholesterol are

- diet
  - some foods are higher in cholesterol than others, or they may contain ingredients that can contribute to high cholesterol
- physical activity
  - physical activity can help raise 'good' cholesterol levels (HDL) and lower triglycerides. Aerobic or cardio exercise and resistance training are particularly helpful for controlling cholesterol levels
- medication
  - your doctor will recommend medication to help lower your cholesterol and reduce your risk of heart attack or stroke. Follow your doctor's advice and take the medication as directed. Do not stop because you feel better. The medication will continue to work in the background to keep your cholesterol under control.

As high cholesterol does not have any obvious symptoms, it is important that your levels are checked regularly through blood tests ordered by your doctor.

high blood pressure

High blood pressure is **the single biggest risk factor** for cardiovascular disease. Even a modest reduction in high BP can have a profound effect on the risk of heart attack or stroke.

Clear recommendations for blood pressure exist. Guidelines issued by many countries around the world, including Australia, say a BP of 130/80 is a reasonable goal for most people with cardiovascular disease. For people who are younger, and who do not have diabetes, evidence suggests 120/70 would be better.

Generally, high blood pressure has no specific cause; however, there are several factors that can increase a person's chance of developing it, including

- family history
- eating patterns (including salty foods)
- alcohol intake
- smoking
- weight
- stress
- levels of physical activity.

Lifestyle modifications are the best way to begin to control blood pressure, including

- eating a healthy diet (less salt, fewer unhealthy fats)
- managing blood cholesterol levels, diabetes, weight
- not smoking
- limiting alcohol consumption
- being physically active
- looking after one's mental health.

Medications are also used.

Obtaining an accurate blood pressure reading, particularly in a specialist's consulting rooms, is not easy to achieve. Often, patients have trouble finding a car park, have had to walk a distance or they worry about what the cardiologist will say, and, perhaps, even what it will cost. By the time of the blood pressure test, the reading could be 'through the roof'.

When a patient's blood pressure regularly goes up while visiting the doctor, it is known as 'white coat syndrome'.

If possible, out-of-office blood pressure measurements are often used. Patients go to their local pharmacy, have their blood pressure checked between visits to their doctors, and write the results in a diary. These, in association with the doctor's measurements, provide a bigger-picture approach that gives the treating medical practitioner a much better idea on the patient's ongoing blood pressure control.

Another option is for the patient to wear a 24-hour BP monitor. The person wears a small machine that is attached to a cuff that measures BP twice every hour during waking hours and once an hour during sleep. Such monitoring gives a detailed profile and information for determining therapy. This monitoring is particularly useful in determining if blood pressure therapy is needed in the first place, and later in the treatment, to ascertain how well blood pressure is being controlled.

The European guidelines say that the 24-hour blood pressure monitoring should be done before initiating any BP treatment, to confirm the patient does have high blood pressure.

Home blood pressure-measuring devices are also popular.

Achieving and maintaining good blood pressure are important in preventing heart problems and in rehabilitation once they have manifested. Long-term high blood pressure on the heart causes structural change which can lead to a person developing atrial fibrillation (AF) and/or cardiac failure (CF). The incidence of both conditions is increasing markedly as the age of the population increases, especially within the Western World. AF and CF are the two most common causes of hospitalisations for people with cardiac problems, having overtaken heart attack.

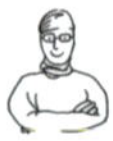

Controlling blood pressure is not as sexy or exciting as having a trip in the back of an ambulance or having a stent put into an artery, but it is the single most useful intervention for long-term cardiovascular health.

obesity

About two-thirds of the adult community are either overweight or obese. This should be a preventable problem in society, yet its prevalence is increasing. Health risks extend well beyond heart disease.

A key issue here for the patient is the driver behind the weight issue.

- Does the person have an eating disorder?
- Is it a lifestyle issue where a poor diet and lack of exercise could contribute to the problem?

If there is an eating problem, the person needs sound education and, maybe, other professional advice. If it's a matter of unhealthy lifestyle choices, then

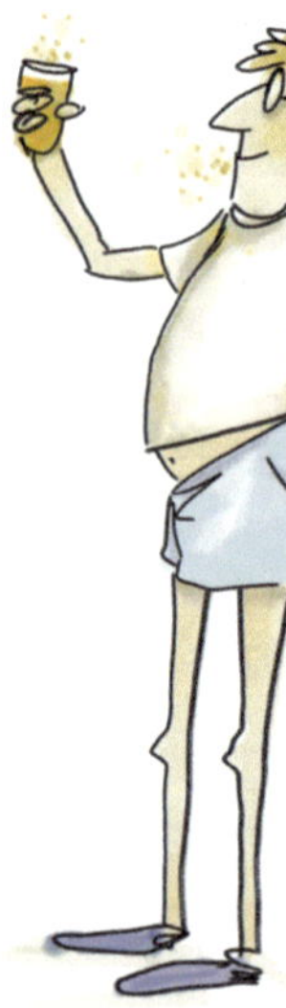

- how much exercise is the person doing, what type of exercise and how often, and
- what are the reasons behind not eating well
  - financial, education, skills, time, interest, ease?

For most people, though, the issue is what and how much they eat.

Dr Bishop has a weight loss program:
https://healthyheartnetwork.com/page/weightloss
also, please see Chapter 12 and Appendix 4

Again, numerous programs are available that can help – from an educational perspective and also from the food planning and preparation standpoint. Other interventions – including medication and, if needs be, gastric surgery – are also available options in more recalcitrant cases. The patient's GP should be involved in these discussions, too.

diabetes

Diabetes adds complexity to the cardiovascular scene. Diabetics do not respond well to standard treatments and their outcomes are worse than for people who do not have diabetes.

Prevention is key, especially averting factors that cause diabetes including

- being overweight
- being sedentary
- having a poor diet.

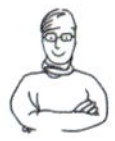

Everyone should have their blood sugar checked regularly by their GP or health care provider.

A class of drugs (sodium-glucose transporter inhibitors, SGLT2 inhibitors), developed in recent years, is providing refreshing news about diabetes and heart disease. The drugs stop reabsorption of sugar in the kidneys by allowing sugar to pass into the urine. When the patient passes urine, the sugar level in the blood is reduced.

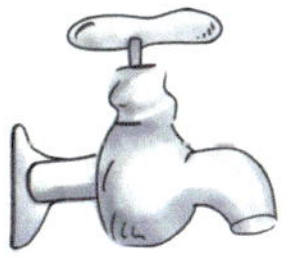

The SGLT2 inhibitors act like a leaky tap of glucose allowing glucose to drip from the body.

Although developed for diabetes, they are effective in preventing cardiac failure and with good benefits for improving blood pressure and weight control. While more studies are being done, use of these drugs is preventing hospital visits and improving patient survival.

When these agents were being tested for their efficacy and their effectiveness in diabetic patients in a trial called EMPA-REG[52], researchers found – to their surprise and beyond explanation[53] – that drugs (such as empagliflozin) were helping patients with cardiac failure.

The DAPA HF study[54], released in Paris in 2019, used the same class of drug (dapagliflozin) with established cardiac failure patients. Both diabetic patients and non-diabetic patients showed equal benefit.

A new frontier for management will open through the use of these drugs. They may be an excellent dovetailing therapy to improve not only sugar control but cardiac function as well.

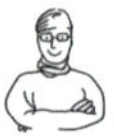

Potentially, they could become drugs for cardiologists to use rather than a drug for diabetes. This is very exciting for the cardiology community.

Dr Alistair:

My experience with using these drugs is very favourable.

Dr Warrick:

They are becoming more available through the Pharmaceutical Benefits Scheme (PBS) in Australia and I am sure will soon be in widespread use. These studies have alerted me to be aware of patients with diabetes and cardiac failure in a new way. It is a research space to be watched and anticipated.

There is also another new class, GLP-1 drugs. The glucagon-like peptide 1 receptor agonists (GLP-1 RAs) act on the incretin hormone system, a system charged with helping the body metabolise carbohydrate. These agents increase glucose dependent insulin synthesis, suppress appetite (through action in the central nervous system), delay gastric emptying and appear to have a positive effect on reducing blood pressure, reducing inflammation, and improving vascular endothelial function.

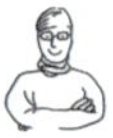

Potentially, this class of agents not only improves diabetic control but also aides in weight loss and control of high blood pressure – all of which are good when it comes to the heart.

stress

Stress is personal and each of us reacts differently. Importance should be placed on knowing stressors and how to manage them. A stressful situation can set off reactions within the body that lead to the heightened 'fight or flight' response.

Positive mental characteristics include happiness, optimism, gratitude, sense of purpose, life satisfaction and mindfulness. They promote health benefits linked to a lower risk of developing heart disease including lower blood pressure, better glucose control, less inflammation within the body, lower cholesterol.

Some ways to mitigate stress are:

- take regular exercise (walking, yoga)
- make time for friends and family (trusted social connections are important)
- have enough sleep (7-9 hours a night)
- adopt a positive attitude
- practice relaxation techniques (meditation)
- find a stimulating hobby
- attend stress management or relaxation classes
- seek a trained healthcare professional for additional support.

Being aware of, and on the lookout for, some of the 'red flags' for **depression** linked to a cardiac event are also important so it may be identified early. Indicators[55] include:

- suffering mental health issues prior to the cardiac event,
- experiencing significant financial strain,
- being younger (aged under 55),
- having poorer physical health prior to the cardiac event,
- being socially isolated,
- suffering a recent bereavement, and
- being a smoker.

It takes a village

Dr Bishop speaks with ROBERT ZECCHIN

president of the Australian Cardiovascular Health & Rehabilitation Association (NSW/ACT) and the recipient of the ACRA Alan Goble Distinguished Service Award in 2021.

Robert is the Nursing Unit Manager – Cardiac Rehabilitation for Western Sydney Local Health District (WSLHD), and an Adjunct Senior Lecturer, School of Nursing, Faculty of Medicine and Health, University of Sydney. He is a clinician-researcher, has been a collaborator on many multidisciplinary research projects and is a published international author[56].

WB **Rob, how would you describe what cardiac rehabilitation is, and the importance of that for an individual passing through the program?**

R *What I believe cardiac rehabilitation to be is an accelerated recovery, both physically and mentally, from a sudden traumatic cardiac event, like having a heart attack, and even a planned bypass graft (operation).*

It's hard to describe the essence of it. It's all individual. The issues that are most problematic are brain fog, with general deconditioning and muscle wasting, pain management, wound management. So, it's someone you need to look after more than others.

Although there's no visible scar involved with, say, a heart attack, you've still got issues about: What do I do now? Is it safe for me to go back to exercise? What do I need to change to promote my life, so I don't have a second heart attack? Will it affect my children and my family? Or my friends? Can they catch it?

WB **So very much providing educational support, obviously, medical support because you've got a nursing background, but also that physical support as well. So, it's a holistic approach, isn't it, guiding people through the other side of a cardiac event?**

R *Exercise is medicine. Everyone's scared of doing some form of exercise or you know,* How am I going to fit that in? *Really, if you've got a pair of good shoes you can walk in (that's all you need). We don't expect people to go into gyms and buy leotards. If you can walk, that's all you really need to do to get and maintain a good level of fitness.*

WB I understand one of your interests is in Aboriginal and Torres Strait Islander people being able to access rehabilitation.

R *About 2004, we piloted an Aboriginal cardiac rehabilitation service, employing an Aboriginal cardiac health worker to be the face of that program to encourage Aboriginal people who have heart problems to come to mainstream cardiac rehab.*

We had evening classes for them and their families because it doesn't affect just that person. If you tell them that they need to go on a certain diet, it's no use telling the guy who's never cooked in his life all about it. You have to invite the partner or the wife, or the girlfriend, or the boyfriend to come along and be educated in that part of the problem area being addressed.

WB It really is very much a village that helps someone recover from these cardiac events. And you're so right. If you don't bring the other family members in or the support people it can fall completely flat. Is the engagement of friends, family, those resource and support people, something that you do routinely through your rehab program?

R *Yes, it's one of the more important components, especially if you have a young, 35-year-old who has had a heart attack, male or female. There's a family history being developed in this situation. So, we must look at the kids. We need to promote healthy lifestyles and surveillance routines in regard to any risk factors they may have as well. Because mum and dad had a heart attack at 35, most likely, if they don't look after themselves – go to their GP, have blood tests, genetic testing – they may also have a heart attack at 35 years of age.*

WB I'm so heartened to hear that Rob, because I see, even with my colleagues who should know better, that they'll treat someone who clearly has a premature issue, but not take the next step and say: *What about your brothers and sisters?* and *What about your kids?* Yet, I think it's our chance to close the loop on cardiac disease and be ahead of the game. I think that's so important; I really do. I'm so pleased to hear of that focus in your unit. Do all units take that holistic approach – not just the patient but the siblings and children as well? Are they proactive in that space?

R *Well, I hope so. But, you know, certain regions have programs that are under-resourced which affects what's available to them in regard to staffing or what time of day they can promote cardiac rehab. Can it be done after hours when people come home from work? Or weekends? That's not to say my program works on weekends, but we do work Monday to Friday. So, we capture quite a large cohort. And we do have some different modalities of cardiac rehab. We have a home walking program. We can provide only education or assessments. We do face-to-face and currently, because of COVID, we do some telehealth as well.*

WB It's an irony to me that there's under resourcing for trying to identify high risk individuals. That's a process that would pay for itself; so, that's terribly disappointing to hear.

On a different note, several unusual conditions occur in cardiology, and sometimes the patients don't get to rehab when perhaps they should. It's an enormously complex topic, but do you want to give us just a few sentences or thoughts around that?

R *One of the most under-populated groups of people coming to cardiac rehab is women. And they have specific types of issues such as spontaneous coronary artery dissection (SCAD) and* Takotsubo *cardiomyopathy, often called stress cardiomyopathy.*

WB Rob, just let me explain.

Rob has described two things, which we see more commonly in women, and generally middle-aged women. One of those things that Rob described is spontaneous coronary artery dissection and that's where the lining of the coronary artery lifts off and tears. It occurs suddenly. It's very scary. It looks like a heart attack, but it's a different process.

And the other thing that Rob mentioned was a condition called *Takotsubo* disease. Now, that's a bit of a mouthful, but it's a particular sort of event-driven change in the way the heart works. Literally, in a big part of the heart, one of the main pumping bits of the heart stops pumping properly. Often driven by huge emotional stresses, it is seen most commonly in women. It's a very concerning condition where people present with shortness of breath and other heart attack-like symptoms. With the right care, it does usually resolve within a few months. Thanks, Rob. Keep on going.

R *A lot of people are scared – even cardiologists are scared – by spontaneous coronary artery dissection in patients. They don't know about exercise components, and the psychological component is huge. Women don't know what they can do:* Can I still hold my baby? Will carrying my baby cause it to tear again? *It's a big issue, and probably more prevalent than we know. But it's something that we are seeing increasingly in cardiac rehabilitation programs.*

WB There are certain conditions that affect women perhaps more frequently than men. If we come back to the run-of-the-mill stenting or bypass grafting, do you deal differently with women and men through the recovery of those?

R *There has been evidence that women-only programs have shown some benefit, but I think it's actually treating the person as an individual... Everyone is different: where they start is different; each heart attack's different; even each stent is different – what type of stent has been used, where it has been put in the heart. Do they have pain or post-stent pain? All these things are individual. I think if we teach or educate the patients individually, it's much better than a generic approach. You are not going to tell a non-smoker about smoking. You do it one-on-one or in a small group in which the patients have very similar issues.*

WB Look that that makes perfect sense. My practice of cardiology is an effort to tailor specifics to the individual. You're saying that rehabilitation is not a production line. You don't just pop someone in one end and pop them out at the other after a sequence of conveyor belt-like interventions. You're meeting those people's needs by figuring out where the needs are and tailoring the program appropriately.

Look in the general scheme of things, how long does a rehab program normally run?

R *Again, that's also individual. It could be as short as four weeks, if that's the patient's preference, but usually its six to 12 weeks, with 12 weeks more for the more deconditioned and older or frail patients.*

WB Do you see the rehabilitation process for stent and bypass as very different? Obviously, the people who have bypass grafting have a huge scar, and they'll never forget the event. Often my patients have a stent and barely skip a beat. What are your thoughts about the rehab process through those different avenues?

R *Well, people who have a coronary artery bypass, as you said, have a scar, and that reminds them every morning about changing behaviours. They're the most so-called 'adherent' population; they are the least likely to drop out. They come to rehab and they don't want to go through that discomfort after the bypass again.*

A stent is a different issue. A lot of patients – and even cardiologists – will say they are 'fixed'. But there is no such thing as a 'fix'. It's a temporary increase of blood flow to a part of the heart. And the patient has to take medication to stop clot formation around the metal stent. And they also need to look at changing the lifestyle behaviours that are detrimental to their heart health.

They tend to be the least likely to stay on programs or come to programs because they've been told they're 'fixed' and they have the attitude: I don't really need to do that. I just need to get back to work and continue on as I am.

If they have a heart attack – a STEMI, or NSTEMI[57] *– it is more likely that they will stay on a rehab program. It's a bit different to just a stent.*

And yeah, we do take them through that education as there is no such thing as 'fixed' in cardiology. There's no cure for coronary artery disease – but we can delay it and people can make healthier lifestyle changes.

WB At times, I almost think we should tattoo a scar on the stent patients just to remind them that we need to continue to care for their heart health; that it is a big thing.

Just before we wrap up, what are the main challenges for the people coming through a rehab program that you identify? And then I'll ask you, what are your main frustrations?

R *So, one of the main challenges is educating the new cardiologists. Sometimes, the new ones are unaware. Sometimes, they are all about imaging or putting in stents, being interventionalist... I would like to see some cardiologists become cardiac rehab specialists. They do in America, and they do in Canada. We've had a few cardiologists involved in cardiac rehab. Have you heard about Alan Goble down in Victoria, who was basically the grandfather of cardiac rehab? He started cardiac rehab in Australia. But they are few and far between. I'd like to see more cardiologists involved in cardiac rehab. But of course, if a cardiologist says 'go', most likely that patient will go.*

My biggest frustration is the referral rates. We would love to see automatic referrals, like referring a patient to occupational therapy or physiotherapy. Refer them automatically to cardiac rehab because they've had a heart attack or a bypass. They will automatically come. If you do that, the resourcing will follow so that the system can cope with the number of patients coming through. Hopefully, the area health service or state government will increase their monies for cardiac rehab.

WB **Look, there's no question in my mind that rehabilitation is incredibly important, and it really does help that whole healing process. And as you talked about, it even starts to close the loop in the community about who might be at risk of heart disease into the future. I really appreciate your sharing.**

As we finish, are there any stories of individuals who stick in your mind that you'd like to share?

R *The patient who comes to mind had an out-of-hospital cardiac arrest. He did a home walking program, completed the program as well and underwent four and six-month checks. Now, he's back on tour. Something that we want for all our patients is for them to go back to what they love best, which includes family, includes their jobs, their friends. And that's what we're all about.*

IMPORTANT POINTS

Change is possible, especially with the help of education.

- **smoking**
  - programs are very helpful when trying to quit smoking
  - general practitioners, in particular, and cardiologists have a role to play in educating and supporting patients to quit smoking
  - stopping smoking effectively reduces cardiovascular risk significantly
  - quitting is a great money saver.
- **physical inactivity**
  - regular exercise
    - > is as effective as an anti-depressant medication for depression
    - > benefits and helps manage heart health
    - > benefits and helps manage other health conditions including some cancers and Type 2 diabetes
  - Heart Foundation recommendation for people 65 years and older
    - > a minimum of 30 minutes a day
    - > five days a week
    - > exercising to a point of moderate intensity
  - exercise includes most movement, including activities that the patient already enjoys
  - physical activity can be increased at any age and from any level of fitness
  - working with an exercise physiologist may be beneficial for many, especially those with diabetes.

IMPORTANT POINTS (continued)

- **worsening cholesterol profile**
  - most cholesterol is produced naturally within the liver and is essential to body health
  - three ways of lowering cholesterol are
    > diet
    > physical activity
    > medication
  - as high cholesterol does not have any obvious symptoms, it is important that levels are checked regularly.
- **high blood pressure**
  - a modest reduction in high blood pressure can have a profound effect on the risk of heart attack or stroke
  - lifestyle modifications can help to control blood pressure
  - medications are also used
  - accurate BP readings are important before starting treatment
  - achieving and maintaining good BP are important in cardiac rehabilitation as a means of preventing another event.
- **obesity**
  - although this is a preventable problem, its prevalence is increasing
  - what is the driver behind the weight issue
    > food choices
      - socio-economic circumstances that lead to the purchase of cheap, poor-quality food
      - lack of education
    > life style
      - poor diet
      - lack of exercise

continued

IMPORTANT POINTS (continued)

- obesity (cont)
  - the most common causes are
    > what a person eats/drinks and
    > how much a person eats/drinks
  - interventions include
    > educational programs
    > medication
    > gastric surgery
  - the patient's GP should be involved in these discussions.
- **diabetes**
  - adds complexity to heart conditions
  - prevention is the key, especially if the person
    > is overweight
    > leads a sedentary lifestyle
    > makes poor diet choices
  - a new class of drugs (sodium-glucose transporter inhibitors, SGLT 2 inhibitors) for diabetes is proving helpful for cardiac patients who suffer cardiac failure, or who experience blood pressure and weight issues
  - another new class of drugs (glucagon-like peptide 1 receptor agonists, GLP-1 RAs) also improves diabetic control, and supports weight loss and control of high blood pressure.
- **stress**
  - as stress is different for each of us, it is important that we know our stressors and how to manage them
  - numerous physical and mental activities are available to help alleviate stress
  - seek professional advice if needed
  - be aware of, and look out for, indicators of depression.

45 *Australia. Each country will have a variety of programs available.*

46 *World Heart Federation website: https://world-heart-federation.org/ What can you do to lower your risk of cardiovascular disease?*

47 *https://www.heartfoundation.org.au/heart-health-education/physical-activity-and-exercise This reference also includes exercise recommendations for other age groups.*

The World Health Organisation updated its Guidelines on physical activity and sedentary behaviour in November 2020. A downloadable publication is available at https://www.who.int/publications/i/item/9789240015128 or a factsheet at https://www.who.int/news-room/fact-sheets/detail/physical-activity

48 *Among the many references to this is one from the Black Dog Institute https://www.blackdoginstitute.org.au/wp-content/uploads/2020/04/5-exercise_depression.pdf which includes sound, practical advice.*

49 *Prince SA, et al (2015) Objectively-measured sedentary time and its association with markers of cardiometabolic health and fitness among cardiac rehabilitation graduates. Eur J Prev Cardiol pii: 2047487315617101. [Epub ahead of print]*

50 *Rogerson M, Le Grande M, Dunstan D et al (2016) Television viewing time and 13-year mortality in adults with cardiovascular disease:*

Data from the Australian Diabetes, Obesity and Lifestyle Study (AusDiab). Heart Lung Circ. 2017 Nov;26(11):e98-e99. doi: 10.1016/j.hlc.2017.03.153. Epub 2017 Apr 20.

51 *2020 International Society of Hypertension Global Hypertension Practice Guidelines*

Thomas Unger et al. originally published 6 May 2020 https://doi.org/10.1161/HYPERTENSIONAHA.120.15026 Hypertension. 2020; 75:1334–1357

52 *Empagliflozin, Cardiovascular Outcomes, and Mortality in Type 2 Diabetes*

Authors. Bernard Zinman, M.D. et al, and Silvio E. Inzucchi, M.D. for the EMPA-REG OUTCOME Investigators November 26, 2015 N Engl J Med 2015; 373:2117-2128 DOI: 10.1056/NEJMoa1504720 https://www.nejm.org/doi/full/10.1056/NEJMoa1504720

conclusions: Patients with Type 2 diabetes at high risk for cardiovascular events who received empagliflozin, as compared with placebo, had a lower rate of the primary composite cardiovascular outcome and of death from any cause when the study drug was added to standard care.

53 *"What was remarkable in that finding was that the benefit was driven by reductions in hospitalisation for heart failure and cardiovascular mortality but not by a lower frequency of myocardial infarction or stroke. Moreover, empagliflozin appeared to slow deterioration in renal function, and the heart-failure benefits persisted in the presence of renal dysfunction."*

Heart Failure Therapy – New Drugs but Old Habits? (editorial) November 21, 2019 N Engl J Med 2019; 381:2063-2064 DOI: 10.1056/NEJMe1912180

54 *Dapagliflozin in Patients with Heart Failure and Reduced Ejection Fraction (DAPA HF study) John J.V. McMurray et al and Chern-En Chiang, M.D., Ph.D., et al., for the DAPA-HF Trial Committees and Investigators November 21, 2019, N Engl J Med 2019; 381:1995-2008, DOI: 10.1056/NEJMoa1911303 (New England Journal of Medicine)*

https://www.nejm.org/doi/full/10.1056/NEJMoa1911303

conclusion: Among patients with heart failure and a reduced ejection fraction, the risk of worsening heart failure or death from cardiovascular causes was lower among those who received dapagliflozin than among those who received placebo, regardless of the presence or absence of diabetes.

55 *Murphy, B. M., Ludeman, D., Elliott, P., Judd, F., Humphreys, J., Edington, J., Jackson, A., & Worcester, M. (2014). 'Red flags' for anxiety and depression after an acute cardiac event: 6-month longitudinal study in regional and rural Victoria. European Journal of Preventive Cardiology 21(9), 1079-1089.*

56 *He has also contributed to the development of the Cardiac Society of Australia and New Zealand (CSANZ) standards for exercise stress testing nationally. He is a member of the National Cardiac Rehabilitation Measurement Taskforce and Chair of the NSW CR Data Working Group.*

Beginning his career as a cardiac nurse in the 1980s, his hospital had one of the first cardiac rehabilitation programs in Australia, and the first one in Australia that promoted exercise stress testing, exercise monitoring, and high-intensity interval training. When he moved on from acute nursing in the early 1990s, he became the program manager of his hospital's cardiac rehabilitation unit.

57 *The difference between the types of heart attack (remember, the medical term for heart attack is myocardial infarction) is determined by the results of the ECG. STEMI stands for ST-Elevation Myocardial Infarction. NSTEMI stands for non-ST-Elevation Myocardial Infarction and while it is the less serious of the two because less damage is done to the heart, it is still a serious condition that requires immediate diagnosis and treatment.*

A certainty comes into your life after a heart event or diagnosis – medications!

chapter 9

AN ARSENAL OF HIGHLY EFFECTIVE DRUGS

Today, health care providers have an arsenal of highly effective drugs at their disposal for treating heart disease and trying to prevent worsening health scenarios for patients. People who have suffered a cardiac event often are prescribed several medications, some of which they will take for a time while others might be for life. Understanding what each drug does and how it should be used safely are keys to successful treatment and prevention that will aid the patient in both quality of life and life expectancy.

Rehabilitation education supports patient understanding and amenability to whatever drug regime lies ahead.

Here we consider the most used heart medications, why they are used, and some of the side-effects to look out for should you be taking them. We also answer the question, *How long do I need to take these for, Doc.?*

blood thinners

There are two main types of blood thinners: **antiplatelets** and **anticoagulants**. The former, such as aspirin, prevents blood cells (platelets) from clumping together to form a clot. The latter, such as heparin, warfarin, and newer agents called non-vitamin K oral anticoagulants (NOACs), slows down the body's process of making clots.

antiplatelets

Let's start with **aspirin** as it is used very commonly in cardiology.

Clots can form within the arteries – the blood vessels supplying the heart and the neck – blocking the artery and stopping the blood flow. Platelets, which are small particles within the bloodstream, are central in the formation of a clot (thrombus). When damage or any abnormality is detected in the inside lining of the artery, platelets become sticky and clump together.

Platelets can be activated often by a rupture in the underlying structure of the blood vessel. Aspirin reduces the stickiness of those platelets, decreasing the likelihood of a clot forming, and so lessening the risk of a heart attack, or even a stroke, occurring.

Because aspirin thins the blood, there is an **increased risk of bleeding** – from the bowel or nose, in the gut (particularly stomach ulcers), or the brain. And say, if you work in the garden and prick yourself with a rose thorn, you may bleed a little longer than usual.

Aspirin can stir up asthma, while other people can be allergic to aspirin, exhibiting swelling and a typical allergic reaction including rash, wheezing, and low blood pressure.

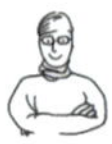

As always, if there are any side-effects, follow up with your GP or specialist, depending on who commenced the medication for you.

Other medications can help with thinning the blood by also making the platelets less sticky. If, for example, you've had a heart attack and you have required a stent, you will be asked to take **clopidogrel**, which is used in combination with aspirin. The two drugs used together is called **dual antiplatelet therapy** (DAPT).

Increased bleeding is the risk with using clopidogrel.

A patient might be on **prasugrel** or **ticagrelor**, which are similar to clopidogrel. These, too, can be used in combination with aspirin for people who have had a heart attack that did not require a stent, but also when a stent has been used.

After a stent has been inserted, a second antiplatelet will be used for about a year. Commonly, clopidogrel will be used, but it could be prasugrel or ticagrelor. These antiplatelet agents can be used in patients who are allergic to aspirin as well. The main side-effect for all of them is risk of bleeding.

A CLOSER LOOK

aspirin

Acetylsalicylic Acid (ASA) is a drug that is known the world over. First registered by the German pharmaceutical company, Bayer, in the late 1800s, the household name by which it is known today, aspirin, was registered in 1899.

For more than 2000 years prior, an understanding existed that something in the leaves of the willow tree and other herbs and plants, most of which contained salicylates (which act like preservatives), had healing properties. The advent of synthetic salicylate acid led to the development of ASA and the marketing of aspirin. Its use has become so widespread that currently it is the most widely used medical preparation in the world, with around 100 billion pills produced each year.

These are almost incomprehensible numbers yet when you stop to think about what it can do the figures begin to make sense.

Aspirin, a non-steroid anti-inflammatory drug (NSAID), works by blocking an enzyme called cyclooxygenase (COX), which leads to the formation of chemical messengers called prostaglandins that cause inflammation, swelling, pain and fever. Altering their production impacts a range of scenarios:

- Prostaglandins within the brain influence the way fevers develop. If you have the 'flu and a fever, taking aspirin blocks your cyclooxygenase, lowers the prostaglandins that are responsible for the fever, and your temperature will drop.
- Prostaglandins have a role in appreciation of pain and the way pain receptors respond. If you have a headache (perhaps with your fever) then blocking your cyclooxygenase and altering your prostaglandin production will ease the pain.

- Prostaglandins also influence the way blood vessels respond in settings of inflammation. If you had a sore arthritic knee from too much work in the garden, the associated swelling could be reduced by again blocking the cyclooxygenase which will reduce the prostaglandins involved in the inflammatory response.
- Another function of the prostaglandins is to protect the lining of the stomach from acid. If you use aspirin for any length of time, the change in the prostaglandins within the stomach may lessen the body's resistance to the formation of an ulcer.

Side-effects from aspirin can lead to possible bleeding within the gastrointestinal (GI) tract. Here, cyclooxygenase-blocking reduces protective prostaglandins, leading to an increased risk of ulcers within the upper GI tract and, therefore, possible bleeding.

This is one side-effect of which we need to be acutely aware when we consider the risks and benefits of taking aspirin in the longer term. A couple of tablets occasionally will not have detrimental effects on the gastric lining; however, ongoing, continued impact on the prostaglandins will.

Still, there are **good reasons** you might take aspirin for the longer term. Aspirin has a role in reducing the stickiness of platelets. Platelets are the small particles in the blood stream involved in the formation of clots. Any irregularity within the blood vessel activates them. Take, for example, a cut; foreign material encountered by the platelets activates the platelets to clump. If they happen to be in an artery, then the clot that forms can block that artery. A ruptured plaque within an artery is the mechanism by which a heart attack occurs when that ruptured plaque exposes tissue factors to the platelets that lead them to clump and form a clot.

The benefit of reducing platelet stickiness in lowering the risk of a heart attack has been demonstrated multiple times since the ISIS-2 trial[58], in 1988, showed that giving aspirin to patients soon after a heart attack reduced the likelihood of that patient having another heart attack compared with not giving aspirin at all.

This first trial has been followed by many others; all of them in the setting of preventing a second event and all of them showing benefit in reducing the risk of a subsequent heart attack. Because of the first heart attack, these patients are all at very high-risk of a second event.

Where controversy has simmered over the years is around giving aspirin to people ***before*** they have an event, that is as ***primary prevention*** before they have declared themselves as very high risk. In recent years, numerous trials have tried to answer this.

In August 2018, a study called ASCEND was published in *The New England Journal of Medicine*[59]. This was a trial that studied patients who were diabetic but had not had any history of heart problems. They were a primary prevention population.

These patients, about 15,500 of them, were followed over seven years. Although there was some suggestion that the risk of having a heart attack was reduced in the aspirin group, this benefit was offset by an increased risk of bleeding caused by being on long term aspirin and the impact that had on the risk of bleeding from the upper part of the gut or into the brain.

Released at the same time but in a different publication, *The Lancet*, the ARRIVE study[60] showed that aspirin had no significant benefit in outcome when given to 13,000 subjects randomised to aspirin or not. These were people with moderate cardiovascular risk but who had not had a previous heart attack or stroke.

A moderate risk means between 10 per cent and 20 per cent risk of an event in 10 years.

These patients were followed for about six years and during that time any benefits in reduction of stroke or heart attack were matched by complications of bleeding.

The most recent was the ASPREE trial[61]. This enrolled nearly 20,000 people across the world (March 2010 - January 2018) to evaluate if aspirin, given to otherwise healthy older adults, over 70 years of age, would improve function and reduce death. There was no suggestion that giving aspirin to this healthy group of older citizens made any difference. There was, instead, a small suggestion that it could worsen outcomes. It is worth noting that these healthy older adults had become healthy older adults because they had not had coronary artery or cardiovascular disease up until then. So, to some degree, the group had been self-selected as a relatively low risk group to benefit from aspirin in the context of reducing cardiovascular risk.

Where does all this information leave us now?

It seems that aspirin should not be used just to try and reduce risk of heart attack and stroke for everyone. It certainly does not have a clear-cut indication in normal primary preventative situations of low or moderate/ intermediate risk patients.

Some data suggest that patients with elevated blood pressure could benefit from being on aspirin. That is probably because elevated blood pressure can push people into a higher risk category.

Dr Warrick:

I like to be more precise in evaluating the risk that an individual may be carrying in the primary preventative setting. I undertake imaging of their coronary arteries. None of the primary prevention studies discussed above incorporated imaging as a selector for aspirin therapy or not. The combination of using imaging and aspirin in primary prevention remains unanswered and speculative. If, on imaging, I find people with high or very high-risk features, then understanding the pros and cons of using aspirin coupled with the individual's situation may lead to use of aspirin as a reasonable consideration. This needs to be approached on a patient-by-patient basis, considering all the available information while striving for the best management strategy for that individual.

In secondary prevention, that is involving people who have had a heart attack or stroke, there remains no question that aspirin is beneficial.

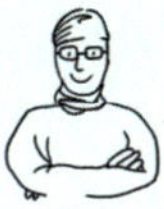

If you have had a problem with your heart arteries, neck arteries or arteries in your legs and you have been prescribed aspirin by your doctor, that aspirin will certainly help. Do not be confused by media reports of the ASCEND, ARRIVE and ASPREE trials. If you have any concerns, please speak with your general practitioner or your cardiologist. Every treatment needs to be based on the merits of benefit of that therapy weighed clearly against any inherent risks. Work with your medical advisors for your own best outcomes.

anticoagulants

Anticoagulants are the other important agents used in cardiology to thin the blood. For example, in atrial fibrillation (AF) thinned blood reduces the chance of a clot forming in the heart.

Anticoagulants work in a different way to the antiplatelet agents, aspirin and clopidogrel and clopidogrel-like drugs. Scenarios where anticoagulants are used include:

- for patients who have had a 'big' heart attack and a clot forms in the heart
- when a mechanical valve has been inserted, and
- sometimes after a tissue valve insertion (for a brief time).

While **warfarin** and **heparin** are possibly the more recognised drugs by name, **non-vitamin K oral anticoagulants** (NOACs) are newer agents that very effectively keep the blood thinner.

Generally, the NOACs act quickly and, so, can be used in an emergency, and they are very well tolerated. The limitations are that the patient

- needs adequate and stable renal function so that the drugs do not build up in the body and cause toxicity problems. Should renal function be a problem, warfarin is the tried and tested option – while it needs to be monitored and adjusted on a regular basis, it works; and
- has no specific heart valve problems. Should the patient have a valve problem, warfarin is the appropriate agent.

Most conveniently, the NOACs do not need regular blood tests to monitor their affect. However, in Australia, specific criteria need to be met for them to be prescribed and funded by the Commonwealth Government under the Pharmaceutical Benefits Scheme. NOACs include the drugs **apixaban, dabigatran** and **rivaroxaban**.

The main side-effect is related to increased risk of bleeding, for example, from the gut or a nosebleed, or, most concerningly, the brain.

Usually, it is much easier to deal with a bleed than it is to deal with a blocked artery or a stroke. You must speak with your doctor if you are having any trouble with your blood thinning medication.

Apixaban and rivaroxaban are very similar although there is a sense within the medical fraternity that apixaban is slightly gentler for the older age group, particularly for people with slight renal impairment. However, practical application suggests that the convenience of rivaroxaban as a single daily dose is preferred by patients. The use of dabigatran also produces similar outcomes for the patient. However, it has a specific **reversal agent** while the other two drugs have a specific reversal agent that will likely soon[62] be available. A reversal agent is significant should the anticoagulation need to be stopped quickly, especially in an emergency. However, each agent can be reversed with the use of blood products in an emergency.

cholesterol-lowering agents

If anyone has had a problem with his or her arteries, that person will almost certainly be taking a cholesterol-lowering agent to achieve the level of cholesterol proven to reduce the risk of future events. Current recommendations are that anyone who has had a stroke, a heart attack, a stent, or a bypass will take cholesterol-lowering medication. Good evidence shows that lowering cholesterol in people who have had an event, and who remain at high risk, can reduce the risk of a future heart event.

The most common cholesterol-lowering medications are the group of drugs called **statins**. Numerous statins are on the market. **Simvastatin** was the first popular agent; then **pravastatin**, which was followed by **atorvastatin**, and, more recently, **rosuvastatin**. These agents are significant in trying to stabilise the plaque within the arteries.

Although most people taking these agents do not experience side-effects, some patients will have problems with the medication. Side-effects vary. The most reported are muscle aches and pains, headaches and nausea.

Report any aches and pains to your doctor. However, it is useful to have an idea of what those aches and pains were like before you started on the medication. Before and after! AND do NOT stop taking medications without speaking with your doctor first.

Another cholesterol-lowering agent is **ezetimibe**, which, when used in conjunction with the statins, offers an extra 20 to 25 per cent cholesterol-lowering ability in people who have very high cholesterol levels. Mostly well tolerated, it can cause some gastrointestinal upset and flatulence.

In very high-risk situations, other newer agents may also be used for lowering cholesterol. This class of drugs acts on a protein associated with a cholesterol receptor in the liver. The drugs are called PCSK-9 inhibitors. Currently, they are expensive and require a specialist to prescribe them.

In 2022, we're in an exciting space in which new agents are on the therapeutic horizon, including mRNA agents (like the Pfizer vaccine) and therapies which work in different places in the cholesterol pathway to the statins and ezetimibe.

ANSWERING YOUR QUESTIONS ?

what is the best treatment for cholesterol?

Some people have very strong – sometimes adamant – views about cholesterol and its role in heart disease, and statins and their role, or not, in preventing heart disease. Such views are often formed from media and Internet opinion. The views are polarised, and the people are clearly passionate about their position. Occasionally, they are fixed and do not allow opportunity for discussion or learning.

Among the strongest held views are that cholesterol is not important in the development of coronary artery disease and that statins do not work and have unacceptable side-effects, including among other issues, loss of memory, cancer, weight increase, depression.

How can such a wide divergence of views be addressed when many patients undertake their own non-medical research and yet there is a large body of medical literature and guidelines that supports the use of lowering cholesterol by treating people with statins?

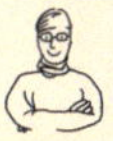

People undertaking their own research is good for their personal education, but they must understand what they are learning and how the information fits together.

A primary consideration here is an understanding of the difference between association and causation. A simple example is a car accident. Speeding and alcohol increase the risk of an accident. Yet, an accident does not occur every time the driver speeds or consumes alcohol before driving. The speeding and the alcohol are ***associations***; they are ***not causative***.

When we consider the heart, people with high cholesterol can live their whole life without having a heart attack. Yet, people with low cholesterol have heart attacks. Studies tell us that if we were to take a group of people with high cholesterol and follow that group for 10 years and take a group of people with low cholesterol and follow that group for 10 years, a comparison would show that the people with a higher cholesterol level have a higher rate of heart attack. ***Cholesterol is an association***, not a causation.

We also know that lowering high cholesterol reduces the risk of heart attack in the future. This, again, supports cholesterol as an association. The body of literature which has been building up over the past 30 to 40 years clearly shows that people who are at high risk of a heart attack have a better result by using medication to lower their cholesterol than not taking medication. High-risk includes having had a heart attack, having a stent, or having had coronary bypass grafting surgery, regardless of the level of cholesterol. In this setting, statin drugs are effective and safe, providing excellent efficacy and outcome benefit.

People who say that cholesterol alone does not cause a heart attack are correct; yet that does not mean that it is not involved in the complex process leading to the heart attack.

What is not clear is the outcome for people in the low-risk category, as cholesterol treatment may not necessarily lead to a significant reduction in risk.

When considering treatment to lower cholesterol, factors that need to be considered include:

- whether the patient is high risk or low risk of having a major heart event
- side-effects
- other risk factors the individual might have, including family history, high blood pressure, if the person smokes or has diabetes, and the amount of physical exercise undertaken by the patient.

For a person who has very high cholesterol yet is otherwise fit and well, some guidelines recommend treatment. However, before treatment, a good discussion with your general practitioner would be advisable with the possible outcome of seeing a cholesterol specialist, a lipidologist, or a preventative cardiologist. Cardiac imaging ascertains if there is a build-up of plaque within the arteries. If there is, treating the cholesterol aggressively is sensible. If there is no build-up, the discussion with the medical practitioners continues to determine a course of action that suits the patient and can achieve best outcome objectives.

beta-blockers

Beta-blockers are prescribed for different reasons. They can be used

- for high blood pressure, although this is not as common a practice as in the past
- after a heart attack, for about 12 months, to help reduce the possibility of a fatal cardiac arrest
- for cardiac failure where the heart is not pumping well – heart failure with reduced ejection fraction (HFrEF).

Beta-blockers include **metoprolol, atenolol, carvedilol, bisoprolol, nebivolol**, and **extended-release metoprolol**. They are well tolerated, overall.

Because they are designed to down-regulate the action of the sympathetic nervous system (the 'flight or fight' response of the body) they can cause people to slow down. Sometimes they can cause fatigue, and the need for afternoon sleeps. Low blood pressure needs to be watched, and people living with asthma who are sensitive to any airway constriction can have problems. Very rarely, but important to be aware of, they can cause depression.

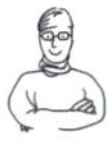

Generally, beta-blockers do a great job.

ACE inhibitors, ARBs

Now let's look at the **angiotensin converting enzyme inhibitors** (ACE inhibitors) and the **angiotensin (AT2) receptor blockers** (ARBs). Both are fantastic medications for high blood pressure or any damage to the heart.

These medications work through the **angiotensin receptor**, providing excellent means of lowering blood pressure by helping the arteries relax (dilate). They can also give helpful changes to the 'hormonal environment' of the bloodstream and assist with the remodelling, or regrowth, of a heart that's been damaged.

These agents are used after a heart attack and to treat cardiac failure.

The first of the ACE inhibitors to be developed, **captopril**, led to improved quality of life as well as improved morbidity and mortality for patients. Since then, several other similar drugs, including **enalapril, perindopril** and **ramipril**, have been developed. The less frequent dosing needed with these newer agents is comfortable and convenient for patients to take and also easier to remember, so less likely to be missed. The newer agents have equal efficacy to captopril.

Commonly used AT2 receptor blockers (ARBs) are **candesartan, telmisartan** and **valsartan**. ACE inhibitors and ARBs can almost be used interchangeably – but not together.

The ACE inhibitors were available before the ARBs and I (WB) tend to use them first. If people have problems with the ACE inhibitors, I change them to ARBs. A potential problem that can be caused by use of ACE inhibitors is cough; that is not the case when using ARBs.

In either use scenario, blood pressure needs to be monitored so that it does not drop too low.

Renal function also needs to be monitored as relaxation of the blood vessels in the kidney can also occur. Any relaxation can lead to a deterioration in renal function. Monitoring requires regular blood tests. Having said that, these agents are commonly used, and they work very, very well.

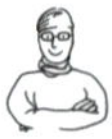

If you've had a problem with your heart, it is common to be on an ACE inhibitor or an ARB. If they cause you any issues, you must let your doctor know.

diuretic therapies

Another class of agents used regularly in cardiology is the diuretic medications. Diuretics lessen the load on the heart by taking fluid out of the body. When the heart is not working properly, it sets off a cascade of chemical reactions that results in the retention of water because of altered kidney function.

A CLOSER LOOK

the kidneys

Our kidneys and the associated urinary system are quite amazing. Together they receive more than a litre of blood each minute and eliminate about 1.5 L of urine each day, effectively ridding the body of excess water and waste products that would otherwise cause serious problems. As blood flows into the kidney, it goes into the glomerulus, the kidney filtration system that filters fluid from the blood. This filtered fluid passes into the collecting tubules which form into a collecting duct that drains into the bladder through the ureters. The collecting tubules – the **proximal convoluted tubule** (near the glomerulus) and the **distal convoluted tubule** (further away from the glomerulus) – have different ways of dealing with electrolytes and fluid. Between the proximal and distal tubules is the **Loop of Henle**. This region is where a further concentration of urine may occur. The diuretic drugs we are discussing act at **either** the distal tubular **or** the Loop of Henle.

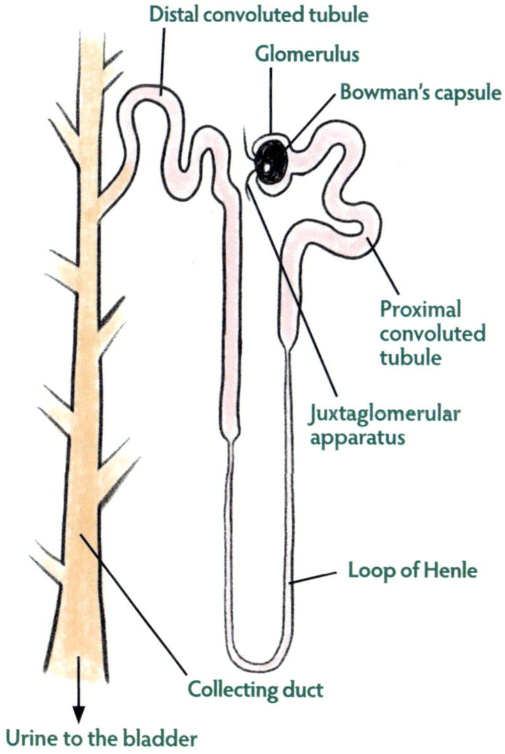

kidney detail

That extra fluid within the body can find its way to the lungs, leading to shortness of breath, or to the body's extremities, such as the legs, where swelling occurs. Diuretic therapy removes the excess fluid and improves symptoms for an individual.

Diuretic therapy comes in three main forms, depending on where it acts within the kidney-urinary system:

- aldosterone blocking agents (in the distal tubule),
- thiazides (also in the distal tubule), and
- the so-called 'loop' diuretic agents (Loop of Henle).

aldosterone blockers

Aldosterone is a hormone that can raise blood pressure and alter sodium (salt) retention in the kidney, which increases the fluid level in the body. Aldosterone blocking agents, or aldosterone antagonists, are drugs that decrease and prevent fluid overload in patients. They work by blocking aldosterone from performing its job of retaining sodium (and therefore fluid) in the kidneys. Blocking aldosterone leads to a reduction in sodium reabsorption, which helps the body pass more water through urine. These are valuable agents for:

- people with raised blood pressure,
- after a heart attack if the patient has HFrEF (where the left ventricle is not pumping as well as it would be in a healthy heart), and
- people in cardiac failure, again, if the patient has HFrEF.

Spironolactone can be a good agent for high blood pressure. Another is **eplerenone**. While they are similar, eplerenone is indicated for someone who has had a heart attack and has reduced pumping action.

Reducing fluid volume may also reduce renal function, so the kidneys need very close monitoring. Both agents, because they alter the function of aldosterone, change the way the kidney deals with the salts, sodium and potassium. Potassium levels can creep up, so the level needs to be checked regularly with blood tests. A potassium level that is too high can trigger dangerous rhythms in the heart. Spironolactone has some crossover with female hormones, and, in men, can cause breast tenderness and breast swelling.

Men, if you are on spironolactone, and have any tenderness around the breast, then it could be from the spironolactone – and you need to let your doctor know.

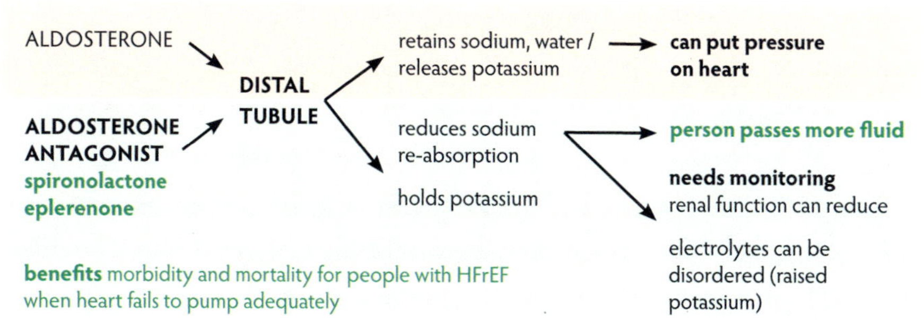

understanding aldosterone and aldosterone blockers

thiazides

Discovered and developed by the pharmaceutical company Merck and Co. in the 1950s, the first thiazide diuretic, **chlorothiazide**, was launched in 1958. Since then, thiazide diuretics have been a mainstay of blood pressure therapy offering an effective, generally well-tolerated, and cheap option.

The thiazides work through two processes.

Firstly, they block the sodium (salt) retaining function of the distal convoluted tubule in the kidney. The resulting salt and water loss reduces blood volume and so lowers blood pressure. The medication, generally taken in the morning to reduce the need to pass urine during the night, often produces a fairly weak effect compared to other diuretic agents and most patients will not notice a significant increase in urine production.

Secondly, they lower blood pressure by dilating (relaxing or widening) the blood vessels.

Imbalance of salts, particularly low sodium, can be a concern and warrants monitoring through blood tests. An imbalance of salts can also trigger gout (ouch!). Other possible side-effects include a rise in blood sugar levels (needs monitoring) and erectile dysfunction, while sun exposure can be an issue for some.

Side-effects can be reduced by using a lower dose and testing patient response.

'loop' diuretics

'Loop' diuretics work by blocking the concentrating mechanisms within the loop of the renal tubule, known as the Loop of Henle. The most used agent, **furosemide** (frusemide) blocks the ability of the kidney to concentrate urine. It is a potent agent for removing large quantities of urine from the body and is particularly useful for patients holding extra fluid in their body (being 'wet') or significantly congested.

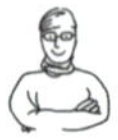

A mineralocorticoid blocker, when used as a diuretic, is often prescribed in conjunction with a loop diuretic. This can augment diuresis as reabsorption of water is blocked in two locations. The doctor then needs to be very careful about fluid balance and fluid loss. Regular blood testing and clinical assessment are essential to ensure the patient is not in fluid over-load or under-load.

As any form of diuretic therapy can also 'dry' a person out too much, they need to be closely supervised. Becoming 'too dry' or dehydrated can shut down kidney function – and that's a problem no-one wants.

Dr Warrick:

For my patients who may need fluid management, I work with them to use the fluid tablets based on agreed criteria reflecting the observations of becoming

- *'too wet', which presents as shortness of breath, swollen ankles and weight gain, or*

- *'too dry', which presents as light-headedness from too little fluid in the circulation, thirst, dry skin and dark urine from an increased concentration of fluid.*

With those triggers, I ask them to increase or decrease the diuretic therapy slightly to adjust the fluid volume and bring them back to the level we want.

Diuretic agents work well. They are reasonably well tolerated. While they don't have many side-effects, they can be inconvenient.

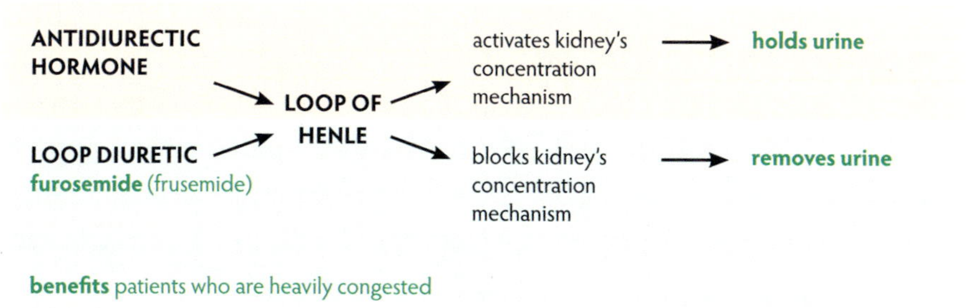

understanding diuretics

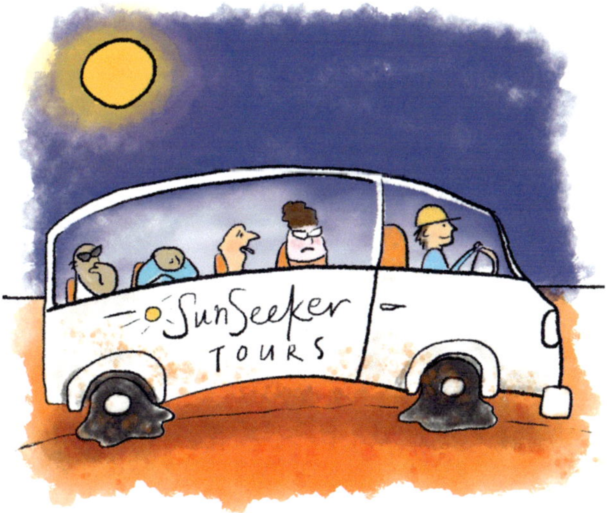

Don't take diuretics before you undertake a three-hour bus trip, or you will have an uncomfortable journey.

sublingual glyceryl trinitrate

Often people are given sublingual glyceryl trinitrate (GTN), which is a spray under the tongue, to be used if they experience chest pain (angina). While it has been used for years, it is given with some caution.

There are two forms of **angina**, stable and unstable.

Stable angina means that the angina hasn't changed for weeks, or even months. You walk, maybe 50m, up a slight incline, and suffer chest pain, and you use the spray. You walk 50m up a slight incline, and feel chest pain, and you use the spray. And this scenario, or similar, is repeated often. There is no question here that GTN spray is effective at alleviating the symptom. However, 50m may be a major compromise of your level of function so, sublingual GTN might **not** be the correct agent for you. You should speak with your cardiologist and ask that something be done for the angina, such as longer lasting agents or even consideration of stenting or bypass grafting.

With **unstable angina**, plaque within an artery ruptures, a clot forms over that plaque and, temporarily, partially blocks the artery. The person feels chest pain, often at rest, and unexpectedly. The person takes a spray under the tongue and that pain goes away. *(Remember Darren Lehmann, page 102?)*

Could there be a problem? What if the person thought the relief from pain was a reassurance that everything was okay *(as Darren did)* and didn't go to hospital *(luckily the ambos over-ruled him!)*?

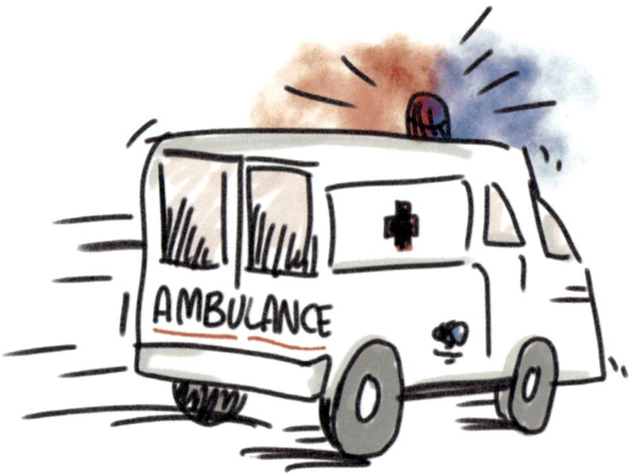

There is no argument to be had. **Unstable angina needs to be managed in a hospital**. So, if a person has the symptom, takes the spray under the tongue and the pain goes away, it can't be left at that. **Use the spray AND call the ambulance.**

Blinding headaches are one of the side-effects of sublingual GTN. Patients need to be aware that the medication can go out of date, although the spray lasts longer than the tablets. Sublingual GTN also interacts with Viagra-type preparations and can cause profound lowering of blood pressure, which can be **dangerous**.

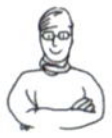

Sublingual GTNs and Viagra do not go together.

BE AWARE!

The sublingual GTN can also mislead. A pain that can replicate heart pain is spasm of the oesophagus. The oesophagus is the muscular tube from the mouth to the stomach that is used for swallowing, and which sits behind the heart. If the muscles of the oesophagus go into spasm, and that can happen if there is reflux, then a spray under the tongue will relax the smooth muscles of the oesophagus. Relief can falsely point in the direction of a heart-related problem when it's the gullet.

nitrates

Nitrates – in particular, **isosorbide mononitrate** – are similar to sublingual GTN. They relax the blood vessels and reduce the load on the heart. However, they work over a longer time so the patient can take them as a tablet and use them as an anti-anginal.

Their use can also result in a blinding headache. If the patient persists with a low dose, building the dosage over several days, the body becomes attuned to it and will tolerate it, without the headache, yet allowing the benefit of the medication. Another side-effect is lower blood pressure. And, again, long-acting nitrates **cannot** be used with Viagra-type preparations.

calcium channel blockers

Calcium causes the heart and arteries to contract more strongly. Calcium channel blockers work by stopping calcium entering the cells of the heart and the arteries. They are used to control blood pressure, chest pain and irregular heartbeat. With cellular calcium uptake blocked, the blood vessels are able to relax and open.

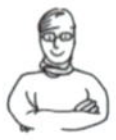

And that's a really nice way to lower blood pressure.

Sometimes, the calcium channel blockers, those called peripherally active calcium channel blockers – including **nifedipine** and **amlodipine** – can cause swollen ankles.

The centrally acting calcium channel blockers – generally **diltiazem** or **verapamil** – can slow the heartbeat. Verapamil can also slow the bowel and may lead to constipation. While it is a good agent for blood pressure and for angina, if constipation results that can be a real problem. Mostly, this bowel problem affects older members of the population, and more often women.

Any calcium channel blocker should be avoided if the patient is suffering cardiac failure.

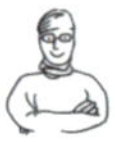

If you have swelling, and you are on a peripherally acting calcium channel blocker, let your doctor know.

for diabetes

The last set of agents are those used in association with diabetes and heart issues. **Metformin** is a good agent which is used for managing Type 2 diabetes particularly in overweight people. Newer agents, particularly the **sodium-glucose cotransporter 2** (SGLT-2) **inhibitors**, are useful for patients with cardiac failure and renal impairment, and the **glucagon-like peptide 1 receptor agonists** (GLP-1 RAs) also appear to reduce cardiac events.

SGLT2 inhibitors block the exchange of sodium and glucose within the kidney, making the patient pass a little bit more urine containing sodium and glucose. Because they help to remove glucose from the blood, it helps to lower blood glucose levels and by removing glucose from the body, these inhibitors can also have benefits for weight loss. Medications include **canagliflozin, dapagliflozin** and **empagliflozin**.

Thrush is the most common side-effect. Care needs to be taken to monitor renal function. Stopping the agents prior to surgery is recommended.

The GLP-1 RA drugs patients may encounter include **semaglutide** and **dulaglutide** – both have the convenience of once weekly dosage – and **exenatide**, which is taken twice daily. These agents tend to result in better blood sugar control than the SGLT2 agents and are the preferred add-on to metformin unless the patient has cardiac or renal failure where the SGLT2 agents have shown clear benefit.

These drugs are generally well tolerated. Gastrointestinal issues are the main reported side-effect. The benefit of reduced appetite and weight loss can't be underestimated in this group of patients.

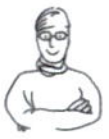

This space of diabetic medications that have a role in reducing cardiovascular risk or cardiac-related outcomes is an exciting one and is currently (2023) advancing in leaps and bounds.

IMPORTANT POINTS

- Understanding what each drug does and how it should be used safely are keys to successful treatment and prevention that will aid the patient in both quality of life and life expectancy.
- Rehabilitation education supports patient understanding and amenability to whatever drug regime lies ahead.

---

58 *International Study of Infarct Survival; Clinical Trial Service Unit and Epidemiological Studies Unit, Nuffield Department of Popular Health (University of Oxford) https://www.ctsu.ox.ac.uk/research/international-study-of-infarct-survival-isis*

59 *Effects of Aspirin for Primary Prevention in Persons with Diabetes Mellitus, October 18, 2018 N Engl J Med 2018; 379:1529-1539 DOI: 10.1056/NEJMoa1804988*

60 *Use of aspirin to reduce risk of initial vascular events in patients at moderate risk of cardiovascular disease (ARRIVE): a randomized, double-blind, placebo-controlled trial Published: The Lancet August 26, 2018 DOI: https://doi.org/10.1016/S0140-6736(18)31924-X*

61 *ASPirin in Reducing Events in the Elderly (ASPREE), Effect of Aspirin on All-Cause Mortality in the Healthy Elderly October 18, 2018 N Engl J Med 2018; 379:1519-1528 DOI: 10.1056/NEJMoa1803955*

62 *June 2022*

Do you want a better, healthier outcome?
Then take your medications.

chapter 10

TAKING MEDICATIONS

Taking medications correctly may seem like a simple or personal matter, but not taking them correctly – or at all – is a common and costly problem. The repercussions can be severe. For instance, not keeping blood pressure under control can lead to heart disease, stroke, and/or kidney failure.

According to the American Heart Association[63], poor medication adherence takes the lives of 125,000 Americans annually and costs the US healthcare system nearly $USD300 billion a year in additional doctor visits, emergency department visits and hospitalisations.

Apart from the health and monetary costs, taking medications as prescribed gives the patient the **best opportunity** to manage a chronic condition and maintain the best possible health. Education, support, and strategies may need to be considered to help patients meet their medication needs.

Education, a thorough understanding of *why I need to take this drug* – often touched on by doctors, elaborated on by nurses in a rehab program and then reinforced by the pharmacist – is extremely important.

Research shows that one of the biggest barriers to patient medication adherence is concern regarding side-effects, so an open discussion about this is crucial.

Cost also could cause a problem. If this is not recognised and addressed early the gains of initial therapy could be lost. A social worker, as part of a multidisciplinary rehab team, can offer support and strategies to meet the patient's needs.

Some patients may need help with organising their lifestyle around the medication or even remembering what to take if there is complexity to the therapeutic regime. Several types of **medication packs** are available. A medication pack can be pre-loaded with the patient's drugs for up to a week in advance to help the patient with dosing and to keep track of what has and has not been taken.

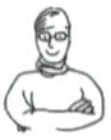

One of my soapboxes is encouraging patients to be responsible regarding the medications they are taking and to always carry a list with them.

Why?

Well, imagine if you are out, fall and lose consciousness. Do you think it would be helpful for your treating doctors at the hospital to find a list in your wallet that lets them know what you are taking – especially if one of those tablets were an anticoagulant? It might just save your life!
So, please, please, please, always have an up-to-date list of medications in your wallet or purse. It will ensure you have the chance of receiving the best health care, especially in the case of an emergency.

Whatever the barrier to ongoing therapy, please raise it with one of the health professionals involved with your rehabilitation, either during the rehab program or in the time afterwards. All of them are working for your optimal health and ongoing enjoyment of life.

"How long, Doc?"

One of the most asked questions in relation to taking medications is: *Do I need to take medications for the rest of my life?*

The answer is simple: *It depends on what heart event you have suffered and the ongoing health of your heart.*

Are you taking medications because you

- have had a heart attack
- suffer from atrial fibrillation or another heart arrhythmia or palpitations
- suffer from cardiac failure
- experience high blood pressure
- have had a stent implanted
- have undergone bypass grafting surgery or
- have received a new valve or have a tight valve?

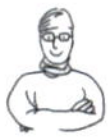

The information that follows is general and must be discussed in detail with your cardiologist and general practitioner or primary healthcare giver.

heart attack

A person who has suffered a heart attack will almost certainly be on a blood thinner such as aspirin, and on a cholesterol-lowering agent as, having already suffered a heart attack, the person is at high-risk of a future event. Both medications will be taken for the remainder of the person's life. Robust evidence says that high-risk patients benefit

- from blood thinning, which makes the blood platelets less sticky and so they are less likely to cause a clot, and
- by lowering cholesterol.

palpitations, heart arrhythmias

Some palpitations may require ongoing therapy; if the patient stops the medication, the palpitations return. Some medications could also treat another problem, such as high blood pressure, and so the patient would be taking the tablet anyway.

If a patient is taking an anti-arrhythmic only for the rhythm disturbance, the problem may be addressed using electrophysiological techniques. Such procedures find where the electrical short-circuit is in the heart and eradicate it.

cardiac failure

Standard drugs for the treatment of cardiac failure (when the heart does not pump properly) include ACE inhibitors, AT2 blockers, beta-blockers and the aldosterone blocker, spironolactone. One of these agents can be swapped for a neprilysin inhibitor. Diuretics are used to move fluid out of the body. While diuretic therapy is not often required long-term, it is very beneficial for relieving symptoms. This therapy can be used on an as-needs basis.

Hearts can recover from cardiac failure. However, about one third of those patients who recover will develop CF again. Standard treatment is that even if the heart recovers, cardiac failure sufferers should remain on their medications long-term.

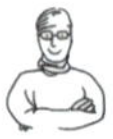

***The management of cardiac failure involves significant complexity. Detailed information is available in my (WB) recent book,* Cardiac Failure Explained.** (See page 295 for further details.)

high blood pressure

High blood pressure is associated with increased risk of heart attack and stroke; it is closely linked to the development of cardiac failure and of atrial fibrillation. When left unattended, it becomes a serious problem. Therapy is for life.

A new technique for treating resistant hypertension, renal artery denervation, is being developed in which the nerves that run along the renal arteries to the kidneys are burned by radiofrequency ablation. Although this can lower blood pressure, generally it is not used as a stand-alone treatment and so, at best, supports on-going anti-hypertensive drug therapy.

stent

If implanted as part of the heart attack treatment, or if received as a preventative measure, the presence of a mesh-like structure in the artery increases the likelihood of a clot forming. This patient will be prescribed an antiplatelet agent in addition to the aspirin and cholesterol-lowering therapy. The patient will be on **d**ual **a**nti**p**latelet **t**herapy (DAPT) for about 12 months, although the time varies according to clinical conditions.

coronary artery bypass grafting

As well as the medication needed for the heart (aspirin and cholesterol-lowering medication, for life), there are several other considerations because of CABG surgery.

The chest wound needs to heal, so antibiotics may be taken for a time, depending on how well the lesion mends.

During the operation, some patients go into the chaotic heart rhythm of atrial fibrillation (AF). They may need to take an anti-arrhythmic agent after the surgery to help the heart return to its normal rhythm.

For most patients who have AF before the bypass grafting, they will need to remain on medication long-term. However, if the AF is permanent (it's not going away) the rhythm medication can be stopped as there is no point in taking a drug to keep the heart in normal rhythm if the medication is not going to have any effect. For patients with AF, the aim is to control the heart rhythm and/or rate and reduce the risk of the blood clotting.

valves

Native valves that leak or are narrowed can be replaced with a mechanical valve or a tissue valve.

When a mechanical valve is used, ongoing treatment includes full-blown anticoagulation to ensure that clots do not form on the new valve, and the patient takes warfarin for the remainder of life.

When it is a tissue valve, the patient will be on

- a blood thinner for a short time and then aspirin ongoing,
- sometimes aspirin immediately following the replacement, and
- sometimes DAPT for a short time and then one agent.

This therapy is very dependent on the individual and the device that has been used. The medication regime requires detailed conversations with the specialists involved.

IMPORTANT POINTS

- Failing to take medications properly – or at all – can have a costly outcome, in terms of both money and health.
- The cardiac event or diagnosis involved and the health of the person's heart are the factors that determine the ongoing need to take medication.
- The need for medications remains a significant and continuing discussion between the patient and his/her medical practitioners.

---

63 *American Heart Association website https://www.heart.org/en/health-topics/consumer-healthcare/medication-information/medication-adherence-taking-your-meds-as-directed*

Are supplements worth considering as additional help?

chapter 11

WHAT ABOUT SUPPLEMENTS?

Often, patients want to know what they can do to improve their health beyond their prescribed medication. While, generally, there is very limited evidence to support the use of supplements being beneficial, the broad use of social media for discussing all things medical means it is almost inevitable that questions about supplements will come up. I (WB) try to be as supportive as possible.

To be clear, this chapter is not an advocacy for supplements and in no way detracts from the proven therapies your doctors will have prescribed for you. However, as the use of supplements might become a topic of conversation with your friends, family or medical providers, here is a little background.

Let's think of these, broadly, as supplements to help with **cholesterol** and supplements that may act as **cardiac tonics**.

cholesterol

bergamot

Some evidence supports the notion that the flavonoids of bergamot, a citrus-based plant, can be beneficial for lowering cholesterol. At least one study[64], undertaken by lead researcher Peter Toth, supports the idea. However, his research was done with a specific proprietary brand of bergamot called bergavit[65].

The study showed that bergamot lowered cholesterol levels (in people who had LDL levels that were moderately elevated) quite well – between 0.5 and 1mmols per litre. The same study also looked at thickening within the carotid arteries (called carotid intima-media thickness[66]). The study suggested that this decreased with use of the bergamot extract.

However, please ensure you have a formulation that is 'good quality' and so likely to work. I (WB) have had patients try bergamot for up to a couple of months. Then, when we have retested their cholesterol levels, the levels have not moved[67].

If you use bergamot – or any other supplement – please do it in conjunction with your doctor, preferably your cardiologist, so there are targets to be aimed for and side-effects, if any, can be mitigated. It is also important that other organs, such as kidneys and liver, are not being impacted.

red yeast rice

Another supplement possibility to reduce cholesterol levels is red yeast rice, a fungus that grows on rice, and contains the chemical from which statins were originally derived. The fungus is used in a natural form and in lowish doses.

World-renowned lipid expert Dr Karam Kostner[68], of Brisbane, Australia, says that the complications he sees with its use are in the reliability of quality and dosage rather than the product itself, which is very similar in chemical composition to a statin.

> *"The problem as I see it is that the production of red yeast rice, which is very popular in the United States, is not as well-regulated as the statins from pharmaceutical companies. The makers do not have to adhere to the same production standards which opens the door potentially to impurities and less active ingredient in the product."*

Side-effects could also be the same as with statins.

> *"If people are prepared to take red yeast rice, I don't see why they wouldn't take a statin. However, if they really want to use it, and are happy with it, I don't have a problem with that approach."*

From a clinical perspective, what is the person's risk and, so, what are we trying to achieve with the person's cholesterol levels? If we are trying to drive down those levels, red rice yeast can be put into the mix and monitored closely.

berberine

Berberine is another supplement that interests my patients. It, too, appears to have a lipid-lowering effect as it seems to replicate, to a small degree, some of the new injectable agents we have for lowering cholesterol that work through the PCSK-9 system.

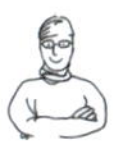

Because bergamot, red yeast rice, and berberine are not what I (WB) routinely prescribe, I ask patients interested in using them to consult a naturopath or other similar expert to achieve the best results.

niacin

Nicotinic acid or niacin is a B-group vitamin that can reduce LDL cholesterol a little; it can raise HDL cholesterol, and it can lower triglycerides a little. Nicotinic acid was used before statins were developed.

The downside is that, as it needs to be taken in fairly large doses, it can cause uncomfortable facial flushing. Based on the HATS trial[69], I (WB) invite patients to try niacin if they need to lower their LDL a little more, or, more specifically, if they have a low HDL and are at significant increased risk.

Although subsequently there have been trials that have shown variability in terms the efficacy of niacin, the HATS trial showed a clear indication that nicotinic acid and statin offered benefit to people with low HDL cholesterol. Although I am still happy to support its use in this group of patients, this agent has fallen out of favour in recent times.

plant sterols

Plant sterols trick the body into not absorbing as much cholesterol as it might. Although they occur naturally in foods such as legumes, vegetables and some fruits, the quantities are not high. Supplements are available in capsule and powder forms and some processed foods are enhanced with them.

policosanol

Derived most commonly from sugar cane, policosanol can alter liver production of cholesterol particles. While some trials have shown that it reduces cholesterol and triglycerides by a small amount, not all studies confirm this. Significant side-effects that impact tolerability can be experienced, and, so, it is not recommended as regularly as other nutraceuticals.

cardiac tonics

Supplementation beyond cholesterol and for heart health generally can be considered in context of

- improving the energy systems of the heart cell,
- the transfer of energy into the heart cell,
- the provision of the building blocks of energy substrate, and
- the provision of energy reaction facilitators.

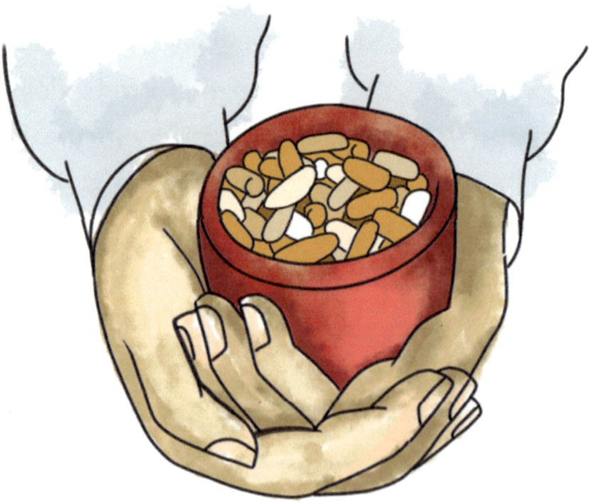

These factors are embraced in Dr Stephen Sinatra's "Awesome Foursome"[70]:

- **Co enzyme Q-10** (CoQ10) is an electron transfer facilitator and can be taken as a supplement. It is possible to measure levels in the blood to guide dosage which can be started at 100mg per day and increased based on need. From my perspective (WB), CoQ10 may have a cellular role in failing hearts. Although some data support this, the studies have not been big enough to draw robust conclusions. However, they have given an inkling that this agent can be beneficial, and I am more than happy for patients to test this for themselves. Theoretical reasons also suggest that CoQ10 supplementation may offset possible statin side-effects, so some cardiologists will suggest it routinely with statin therapy.
- **L-Carnitine** helps the fatty acids get into the mitochondria so they can be used as an energy source. One to two grams daily will support this.
- **D-Ribose** at five grams per day will help provide the building blocks for the energy molecules the heart uses, adenosine triphosphate (ATP).
- **Magnesium** is a co-factor in hundreds of reactions that occur within the body and particularly in energy generation in the heart. Magnesium will also help with blood pressure control and leg cramp. Start at 200mg per day and adjust as needed.

Other supplements include **fish oil**, in which the omega-3 fatty acids, eicosapentaenoic acid (EPA) and docosahexaenoic acid (DHA), are the active ingredients. At times, fish oil is in favour, and at other times, not. According to Dr Kostner, EPA and DHA are excellent for lowering triglyceride levels and for brain development.

Study results are more confusing in relation to sudden cardiac death, cardiac failure and general cardiac conditions. However, one trial, called REDUCE-IT[71], looked at the role of high doses of fish oil (EPA only) given to patients who had a high risk of heart attack, and high triglycerides. It showed a clear benefit.

While there are few side-effects, users need to be aware that many preparations of fish oil are commercially available. When considering purchase, it is wise to check the amount of EPA and DHA in the preparation. A dose needs to be 2 –4 grams of active ingredient. Cheaper brand capsules might contain 300mg, with higher quality brands about 1g. Liquid fish oil can have up to 1000mg /1mL.

Fish oil is the nutraceutical mostly commonly used in Australia.

needs vs treatment manipulations

Dr Warrick:

What we are trying to determine is the patient's treatment needs balanced by the medications and/or manipulations put in place.

In high-risk patients, I want LDL cholesterol lowered as much as possible. Statins are the most widely available and cost-effective way to do it, and, for most people, they work well.

As with all supplements, issues of their efficacy, cost, and quality exist. My approach is to discuss these options with patients who are interested, and try the supplements under supervision, with an assessment of the effect. I encourage the use of reliable, quality compounds to see if there is a measurable wellbeing benefit to justify the cost. If there isn't, we focus on lifestyle factors and proven medications.

IMPORTANT POINTS

- While not much evidence supports the use of supplements being beneficial for cardiac patients, there are possibilities worth considering. Discuss with your doctor.
- Efficacy, cost, and quality are parts of the equation.
- Supplements do not replace drugs.
- Supplements should be used only under medical supervision.

---

64 *Bergamot Reduces Plasma Lipids, Atherogenic Small Dense LDL, and Subclinical Atherosclerosis in Subjects with Moderate Hypercholesterolemia: A 6 Month Prospective Study Peter P Toth et al PMID: 26779019 PMCID: PMC4702027 DOI: 10.3389/fphar.2015.00299 https://pubmed.ncbi.nlm.nih.gov/26779019/*

65 *As far as Dr Bishop is aware, this extract is not available in Australia.*

66 *used to diagnose the extent of carotid atherosclerotic vascular disease*

67 *This might mean that we were not using a preparation that was effective – see Peter Toth comment on the previous page*

68 *a Healthy Heart Network podcast (ep 137) in which Dr Bishop speaks with Dr Kostner about supplements and nutraceuticals for lowering cholesterol*

69 *HDL-Atherosclerosis Treatment Study – HATS. Date published: 01/01/2001; date updated:05/09/2002. America College of Cardiology. https://www.acc.org/latest-in-cardiology/clinical-trials/2010/02/23/19/07/hats*

70 *Heart MD Institute. Awesome Foursome: Targeted Supplements for the Heart https://heartmdinstitute.com/diet-nutrition/the-awesome-foursome/*

71 *Cardiovascular Risk Reduction with Icosapent Ethyl for Hypertriglyceridemia, Deepak L. Bhatt, M.D., M.P.H., et al. for the REDUCE-IT Investigators* January 3, 2019, N Engl J Med 2019; 0:1122, DOI: 10.1056/NEJMoa1812792*

Medications may help keep you alive, but what are you prepared to change so that you can really live?

chapter 12

NUTRITION FOR LIFE

Poor diet is a leading risk factor for heart disease. The quality and quantity of food eaten, and drink consumed, significantly contribute to the health of a person's heart by impacting several heart disease risk factors including

- high blood pressure
- cholesterol
- weight, and
- the risk of developing diabetes.

There is a widespread misconception that most Australians eat a healthy diet when most are not meeting the Australian dietary guidelines.

Healthy eating involves food that is unprocessed, naturally low in unhealthy fat, salt and added sugar, and rich in whole grains, fibre, vitamins and healthy fat. Fresh and unprocessed products are the best. Small changes that can be continued long-term are advisable, keeping in mind that it is the overall combination of food and drinks over days, weeks, and months that counts.

The heart does not like fad diets.

6 key elements

Six key elements of a healthy-living eating pattern are:

1. **plenty** of
    a) whole fruit (not canned or juiced),
    b) vegetables, and
    c) whole grains;
2. a variety of **healthy protein**
    a) especially fish and seafood,
    b) legumes (such as beans and lentils),
    c) nuts and seeds,
    d) a small amount of egg and some poultry, and
    e) if choosing red meat ensure that the meat is lean, and limited to 1-3 times a week;
3. **dairy** can include
    a) unflavoured milk,
    b) yoghurt, and
    c) cheese;
4. **healthy fat** choices using
    a) nuts,
    b) seeds,
    c) avocados,
    d) olives, and
    e) their oils for cooking;
5. **herbs and spices** to flavour the foods instead of adding salt, and
6. the best choice of drink is **water**.

A healthy-eating plate starts with unprocessed food and consists of one-quarter protein, one-quarter carbohydrates, and one-half vegetables.

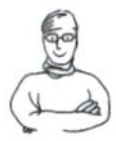

People with high cholesterol and/or diabetes are advised to seek further advice.

PLEASE EAT MORE VEGGIES!

The (Australian) Heart Foundation wants people to eat more vegetables. Staggeringly, more than 90 per cent of Australians do not eat the recommended five serves of veggies a day. Adding just one extra serve to a person's daily intake has heart health benefits.

If all Australians met the vegetables target, it could cut the risk of cardiovascular diseases by about 16 per cent and save $1.4 billion in health spending.[72]

cooking at home

One way to increase fresh produce intake and decrease processed foods is to cook at home more often. Purchased meals and snacks can be high in kilojoules, salt, sugar and unhealthy fats that are often 'hidden'.

Planning ahead, using leftovers in interesting ways and making your own condiments including salad dressings and sauces are also useful tools. The healthiest oil for salad dressings and low-medium temperature cooking is olive oil.

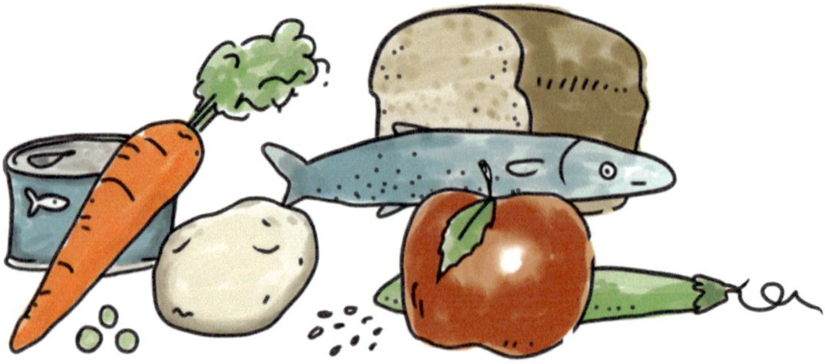

top 5 tips[73]

1. **Aim for 5 servings of vegetables a day**. Add vegetables to salads, soups and casseroles or try them as a snack.

2. **Go for grain**. Replace white bread and rice with wholegrain and seeded bread, brown rice and high fibre breakfast cereals.

3. **Eat more legumes** like lentils, chickpeas and beans. Use dried and cooked or canned varieties either alone or add to dishes to reduce the amount of meat.

4. **Aim for 2-3 servings of fish a week**. Canned fish in spring water or olive oil can be used; avoid those canned in brine.

5. Try introducing **at least one meat-free day a week**. You can find lots of quick and tasty meat-free recipes at this website: heartfoundation.org.au/recipes

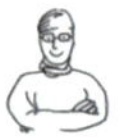

IMPORTANT: Look at the whole plate. Eggs served with spinach, mushrooms and wholegrain bread, for example, will be a better choice than eggs with bacon and white bread.[74]

reading food labels

Nutrition information panel and ingredients lists are good ways of comparing similar foods so you can choose the healthiest option. Almost all packaged foods are required to display a Nutrition Information Panel (NIP) that must meet government standards. The panel is usually located on the back or side of the product packaging. Panels always list

- energy (kilojoules)
- protein
- fat (total)
- saturated fat
- carbohydrate (total) sugars
- sodium.

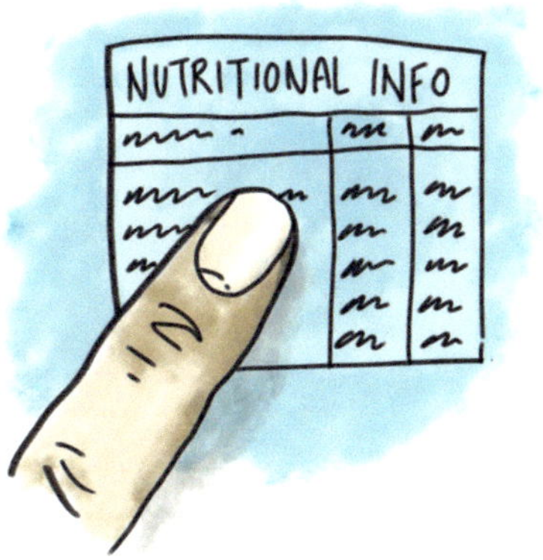

Other nutrients such as vitamins and minerals, fibre and other types of fat may also be listed.

When comparing products, look at the food as a whole rather than deciding based on just one nutrient alone. The quantity per 100g or 100mL column is best when comparing different brands of similar products. Per serving values vary depending on the type of food and the brand. It doesn't necessarily mean you eat the serving size specified on the pack.

fat – Use the 100g or 100mL column to compare similar products to choose the option with less saturated or trans-fat – the unhealthy fats. Trans-fat is often not listed on the nutrient information panel. Avoid foods with 'partially hydrogenated' vegetable oil or vegetable fat, animal fat, copha and palm oil listed in the ingredients list.

salt – Salt will be listed as sodium. Use the per 100g column to compare the sodium content of two similar products. 'Low salt' means less than 120mg of sodium per 100g. Check the ingredient list for other names for salt such as sodium, monosodium glutamate and vegetable salt.

swap this for that[75]

potato crisps	unsalted nuts and seeds air popped popcorn – try adding spices or chilli flakes instead of salt and butter
hot chips	home-made sweet potato wedges (toss wedges of sweet potato with olive oil and bake @180°C for 20-30 minutes)
sweet biscuits and cakes	home-made versions *see recipes at* www.heartfoundation.org.au/recipes/category/baking
fruit yoghurt or ice cream	natural yoghurt with added fresh or frozen berries
ham sandwich	cheese and salad sandwich on wholemeal bread
meat pie	chicken and salad wrap
cream cheese, cheese spread, cheese sticks	mozzarella, edam, cheddar, cottage and swiss cheese
salt	herbs, spices, pepper, garlic, chilli or ginger
soft drinks, fruit juice or cordial	water, mineral water or sparkling water – try adding lemon, lime or orange slices to flavour the water without sugar

For further information on healthy eating, search the websites of various heart-related organisations, for example, "How to Eat Well for a Healthy Heart", on the Heart Foundation website, https://www.heartfoundation.org.au/

IMPORTANT POINTS

- The quality and quantity of food eaten, and drink consumed impacts several heart disease risk factors including
  - high blood pressure
  - worsening cholesterol levels
  - excess weight, and
  - the risk of developing diabetes.
- Enjoy a wide variety of foods ensuring they are
  - fresh and unprocessed produce,
  - rich in whole grains, fibre, vitamins, minerals, and healthy fats, and
  - low in salt, added sugar and unhealthy fat.

---

72 *Heart Foundation media release, 8 January 2020; https://www.heartfoundation.org.au/media-releases/what-to-eat-in-2020*

73 *ibid.*

74 *For some practical recipes, see appendix 4 or visit the website of your country's Heart Association, such as www.heartfoundation.org.au/recipes in Australia*

75 *The Heart Foundation website https://www.heartfoundation.org.au/getmedia/d9ca1d68-fdb3-4efe-9716-5dfeb2802c1e/Eating-well-to protect-your-heart.pdf*

Exercise is one of the critical components for full recovery – and remainder-of-life health and well-being.

chapter 13

EXERCISE

INTERVIEW

A journey of restoration

Dr Bishop speaks with Angela Hartley

a cardiac rehabilitation nurse who trained as a cardiac nurse in Australia and now runs a cardiac rehabilitation service in the United Kingdom.

WB Tell me how your training led you towards cardiac rehabilitation.

A *I did all of my nursing training in Australia, always in cardiac, which I loved even as a student. Just did cardiac, cardiac, cardiac. Worked in Brisbane, in one of the big hospitals there. Then, I moved to the UK for a little working holiday. While I was waiting for my nursing registration over here, which takes about a year, I worked in a gym. I had never previously worked in a gym. (At the time) it was just an easy way to get going in the UK. Then when my registration came through, I worked in cardiac wards for a few months, and then into ICU and recovery. Always in cardiac. And then after a couple of years of doing that, a job came up in cardiac rehab and I thought,* Why not combine the two? *The combination of the exercise and the nursing is the perfect job for me.*

WB I understand that you're now running your own cardiac rehabilitation business. What's your passion about this area of medicine?

A *Well, the reason I set up the cardiac rehab business is I found there was a real gap when people went home from hospital after a cardiac event. So, if they've had a heart attack or a pacemaker put in, or any cardiac surgery, there was this big void. Whilst many people in the UK are entitled to cardiac rehab, which is once a week for between* *six and eight weeks, I found that they felt really left out in the wild, and they didn't have a support network afterwards. I'm trying to fill that gap and give people the confidence to carry on after their state-led cardiac rehab, to carry on with exercise and to get back to doing normal activities and feel really good about themselves. So, I'm really passionate about getting people that confidence back, in particular with exercise.*

WB It's easy to return to old habits that may have got them to the wrong place in the first place. Do you find that these regular visits are useful for not only moral support but accountability to help people stay on the right path?

A *Absolutely. I've become part counsellor, part friend, part slave driver. So, you know, it's sort of mixing them all together to say,* Right, you have to turn up at least once a week. *Some people do more often; some people do less often and then they're just checking in with me every now and then. I have a little homework book for them and I fill it in with what I'd like them to do throughout the week. Depending on the stage they're at, they might just need to do a 10 minute walk every day. For other people that might be, you know, significantly harder than that, depending how far down the line we are.*

Accountability definitely helps as does having someone be your cheerleader to check in on you every week. It gives the person the opportunity to say, Oh, you know, this happened this week. What should I do next time? *or* I was walking up a hill and I felt breathless. Did I go too fast? What should I do next week?

WB Do you find within the groups that there is a lot of interaction between the individuals participating? Do they support each other? And is that a valuable component of rehab to your way of thinking?

A *At first, I didn't have that component and it was all one-to-one work. People really loved that, they benefitted, and they felt listened to. However, once we were a few weeks or months down the line, I felt that group element was missing. So, I set up a local group. We meet once a month; between 20 and 30 people a month. They come, have a chat and a cuppa, and then I give a speech about a different topic, and I try to get guest speakers along every month as well.*

WB That's fantastic. A nice cuppa with 20 or 30 people on a regular basis sounds like a good get-together.

A *Exactly. It's like such a nice place for them to chat about, you know, all their medications and 'this has happened' and 'my doctor said this'. We're not giving medical advice, but it is an opportunity for people to have a chat about their problems because sometimes the family doesn't understand.*

WB I imagine that, for individuals, it must be nice to know that they're not alone travelling this particular path. So, there's strength from others' experiences, and, surely, the interaction gives support both ways.

A *Yeah! There's moral support as well. We've got a guy who is now running 10kms every week. And, he's our inspiration. Some are at the beginning of their journey and he's, obviously, quite far down the line. Listening to people speak about how they've been through so much helps others believe there is another side and that they, too, can come out stronger, and do more again.*

WB One of the things that intrigues me is how men and women are affected by cardiac disease. In your experience, do you think that men and women travel different journeys?

A *I'd say they are different. It depends, personality to personality, and how they got to the place that they're in. Having said that, I find that the men are sometimes a bit more pragmatic, sort of* Tell me what to do, and I'll do it. *The women may need emotional support, encouragement. They may not have exercised for many years. Because they've been looking after families, they didn't have the time. And they may have never prioritised their health. Sometimes, it's getting the women into the healthy habits, and that can be a challenge because they're still looking after grandkids or kids or working.*

In terms of the differences in their journey, I feel the men tend to blame – I've been drinking and eating and not exercising for a few years – *whereas the women tend to be more shocked that they have this diagnosis.*

WB My experience is similar. Blokes will put up their hand and recognise where they may have strayed off the healthy path. I also see men display depression after their events, more obviously, than women. Men seem confronted by their inability to take on the world and I think that knocks them emotionally.

A *I feel like having me as that ear – like I said, I often turn into a counsellor – that's often more the men because they don't want to worry their wife or their children or their even their work colleagues, but here (in the rehabilitation community) is a safe space to open up and say,* You know what, I'm quite scared and I'm not so sure about myself anymore. *It helps build them back up again.*

WB A priority for me is seeing the 'significant other' so that we have everyone on the same page. In your rehab, do you engage the partners?

A *Engaging the partner is a great idea. I get them in at the initial assessment, if they are both happy to come along, but then during the exercise not so much. Then, it is only if the partner really wanted to, or if the partner was worried about things and wanted to check in and make sure it was a safe environment.*

When it comes to the monthly support group, a lot of partners come. They like to meet other partners. They like to have a chat. They like to ask me lots of questions. They like the reassurance that, Oh, you know, this seems a safe space and she knows what she's talking about.

WB Perfect. A win all round!

Another facet that intrigues me is the rehab from two very common interventions, one is stenting, and one is coronary artery bypass grafting. I'm interested to know if you see any differences or similarities after an individual's had stenting (minimally invasive insertion of a small structural device that holds open the blocked artery) or bypass grafting (major surgery that replumbs the artery).

A *We'll start with the similarities as patients usually get referred to their NHS, which is our health system rehab, after about six to eight weeks, although, often by the time they get there, it might be slightly longer. And, so, they turn up about the same length of time after their* *procedure, whether it has been a stent or a bypass. All patients do the same sort of exercise, they hear the same talk and they do the same heart rate monitoring.*

As I always start with an assessment, that would be the same for both sets of patients. This is a little exercise test, and then tailor the exercise as appropriate. In building them back up, I like to say it's a fitness pyramid. The very foundation of that pyramid is their walk. In both groups of patients, I get them doing more walking, building that up gradually. Then, we add the harder exercise as we go, getting gradually more difficult.

In terms of the differences, it depends person to person. However, the bypass patients tend to have more pain and more fear around using their upper body and they experience more discomfort in terms of moving around. They are also a lot stiffer in that their shoulders droop forward as a protection mechanism. As they may have to sleep in a chair or in a recliner chair, they have more postural issues. We do have to work on that, and, then the confidence to use their upper body, again. Obviously, we start gently, and we move on as the weeks progress.

With the stenting patients, because they can't see the stent, theirs are more psychological issues. They can't see that they've been fixed. With the bypass patients, they have an I'm safer with exercise because I've been fixed *attitude although they need to deal with the pain, discomfort, and the lack of sleep. The stent patients ask,* Who am I? I'm okay, but can the stent collapse? Is it really in there? What about the arteries they didn't stent? *So, I feel like the psychological issues are more on the stenting side.*

WB I see similar responses from my patients, too. The magnitude of the intervention is significant. A cardio-thoracic surgical procedure is a big deal. My observation is that those patients are likely to change more to ensure it doesn't happen again, whereas I have some patients who are guilty of breezing in with a whiff of chest pain. They get a stent, and they're back on the road thinking that not much has happened. They don't realise they went very, very close to the edge of the cliff, and then walked away from it.

A *That's a good point as well. Sometimes, that is down to the doctor. A lot of people don't have that fear put into them although they need to change. There's only so much that someone will do with me telling them. Sometimes people can be a bit more lackadaisical about it.*

WB It's a tricky one. You don't want them fearful, but you also don't want them complacent. Before we finish, are there three aspirational goals, or three golden rules you have for your rehab patients, Angela?

A *Yes.* ***Number one is to go slower than you think****. By that, I mean I want you to be a tortoise, not the hare. People say,* I'm getting breathless and feeling tired. I can't do this anymore. *And I say,* We'll do it slower. *This can be frustrating, yet often by doing things slower, and stopping to smell the roses before you keep walking, that will gradually build up a person's fitness. So, always go slower than you think you should and even if you're already slow, go a little bit slower, still.*

Number two is to take one step at a time. *Don't worry about the end goal. This could be about whether you want to lose weight, whether you need to get fitter, whether you want to get back to work. You've got to take one step at a time and think about what you need to do today. That might be your 10-minute walk, which might be next week's 15-minute walk and the week after, a 20-minute walk. But, for today, just worry about today, and so, one step at a time.*

Number three is to get some support. *Have a really good support network with someone like myself, who you know is in your corner who says,* Come on, you can do it. Let's try something else this week. Let's do a little bit more. *It could be a partner; it could be a friend who's a walking buddy you meet up with every week; it could be the dog that drags you out for a walk. Getting some support is key to keeping you motivated and keeping you accountable.*

WB I like that. And finally, Angela, do you have a great cardiac rehab story that you can share?

A *One of my guy patients had full open-heart surgery, an aorta repair together with bypass. It was an emergency, and he was very shocked by it. He was rushed off to hospital, woke up in intensive care, spent a good week in hospital, went home, did the NHS rehab and then sort of fell off the rehab. Like I was saying, there's not that much support after you finish those classes. So, medically, he was quite stable, and his doctor had said he could go back to work if he wanted to, but things weren't right mentally. He had lost his confidence. His family said he was cranky all the time. So, he came to see me. He was probably about four months post-surgery by then.*

A lot of what we worked on was his confidence. Whilst he'd been trying to do some walking, like I said in my tips, he'd been going off quite fast. He'd put the trainers on, out the door, get to the end of the street feeling quite knackered, and ended up going home feeling depressed.

I said that he needed to slow down. My first tip, slow down, and you'll be able to get to the end of the block, and then come home, and then the next week, the suburb, and so on. We built it up more slowly than what he probably thought he should be doing. By going slower, though, he was able to go much longer.

Secondly, we worked on his mindset. He was afraid. This was not something he said out aloud. When we got to the bottom of it, it was, I'm afraid that I'm this old man who's not going to be able to contribute anymore. *Arriving at that point took a lot of work and he was also working with a counsellor during this time. The key was working on his mindset to say,* Look, you are still funny; you've got plenty to contribute.

He went back to work. We had to encourage him to go out with friends again to get his old personality back. And just the realisation for him that he wasn't a write-off. I think that was really key, to be able to say, Hey, there's still plenty you can do, plenty you can contribute.

So those first few months, I think, were crucial for him getting his confidence back. Now, we're doing lots of fun stuff. We're doing boxing every week. We're doing some resistance exercises. He's loving his walking. He's doing 12,000 steps a day whereas previously he hated walking, hated exercise.

I think that was massive progress. The key is that we took it slowly. He listened. He did the homework. Gradually, he walked further and further each week. And now he's got his confidence back.

WB He is a perfect example of how surgery isn't the total fix. It's only the beginning of the restorative journey to health. Angela, you've continued that therapeutic journey for this man to a beautiful outcome.

progressive, structured approach

A progressive increase in physical activity through a supervised and structured program is the best way to approach exercise, or a return to exercise, following a heart event. Healing after a heart attack or any serious injury to the chest takes about six weeks for the muscle to mend and the bones to knit together. During this time, the patient gradually returns to normal activities.

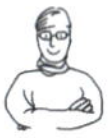

The type of intervention and the damage to the heart muscle determine the length of recovery.

This can be much quicker, depending on the actual procedure that has been done. For example, in stenting, injuries to the wrist or to the groin are minimal – a simple puncture site – and the procedure around the heart to the artery(ies) is, remarkably, minimally traumatic. That patient might resume normal activities within days of the procedure.

At the other end of the scale is the high impact situation in which the person may have suffered a significant heart attack resulting in damage to the heart muscle. The patient might need open-heart surgery to bypass diseased arteries and restore blood flow or replace a valve. This is a big deal.

This is a double whammy because not only is the person recovering from the injury to the heart and waiting for the drugs to improve heart function, but the patient is also recovering from a significant injury to the chest wall and potentially the arm or leg from where the surgeon has taken the graft vessel.

Remember from our earlier discussion: In coronary artery bypass grafting (CABG) the chest is cut open through the sternum (breastbone), and blood vessels (taken from another part of the body – usually arteries from the arm or chest, or veins from the leg) are stitched into the arteries above and below the trouble spots to bypass the narrowed or blocked areas and restore blood flow to the heart muscle. One or more blood vessels may be used, depending on the severity and number of blockages.

Such surgery would be followed by significant recovery and rehabilitation and may take longer than six weeks for the person to resume full activities, depending on the person's age, general health and the complexity of the operation.

It is important for patients to look after their wounds following the surgery. While the patient may feel very well again after six to eight weeks, it can take up to three months for the sternum to heal completely. Patients are advised to take life gently during that extended time, as the last thing they need is to disrupt the healing process.

About two to three per cent of patients develop a 'clicky' sternum, in which the bones, for numerous reasons, don't knit together. This, sometimes undiagnosed, condition is corrected by the procedure, chest wall stabilisation.[76]

Damage can also be caused by something as simple as a cough or sneeze. People recovering from heart surgery, particularly in that first six to eight weeks, should have a pillow nearby so they can hug it during more strenuous movement. The wound is held together by strong wires as the bones are healing. Hugging the pillow stops the wound from shifting.

Additionally, such serious surgery has a psychological impact, and so mental reconditioning also needs to be considered.

how much?

The question now becomes, *How much exercise should a person undertake?*

As we have seen earlier, the Heart Foundation (Australia) guidelines recommend that people 65 years and older with heart disease should accumulate a minimum of 30 minutes of exercise a day, preferably on all days of the week, exercising to a point of moderate intensity (heart rate rises but not to a point of breathlessness). Balance and flexibility exercises should be incorporated on most days and specific strength exercises should be done on two-to-three days of the week. The recommendations also suggest that people do not sit for too long and if new to exercising, should consult their doctor, start at an easy level, and gradually build up.

In rehabilitation, however, the amount and type of exercise depends on how sick and how fit the person is. Consideration needs to be given to the impact the exercise is having on the person rather than saying the person needs to exercise with so many metres or so many minutes.

An exercise program should be tailored for the individual. Such a program is based on what's called a 'perceived level of exertion' or the Borg Scale which is based on the feeling of how hard it is to breathe. Someone who is really struggling to breathe might be at nine or 10 out of 10 and someone who doesn't feel puffed at all might be one out of 10. About six to seven is regarded as 'moderately breathless' and this is the level aimed for in cardiac rehabilitation. For one person it might be a gentle walk, for another it might be running on the spot. Whatever the level, the person possibly does not want to be lifting heavy weights or cycling up hills in the early months of recovery as such strenuous exercise increases blood pressure and puts too much stress on the heart.

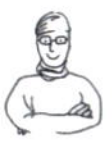

Exercise needs to be individualised as it is more about the impact it is having on the individual rather than any predetermined numerical measurements. Even so, a patient needs to push a personal limit to build personal fitness. Professional guidance is strongly recommended.

Heart illness causes a certain amount of de-conditioning. Aerobic activity, such as walking and low-intensity cycling, is highly recommended for the heart's recovery. The surgery, hospitalisation and sometimes medications contribute to muscle weakness in the arms and legs and, so, muscle-strengthening is also recommended.

If a patient has trouble getting out of the chair, or the person's muscles are feeling extremely weak, this should be mentioned to the cardiologist.

Cardiac rehabilitation exercise programs can be perceived as low-level movement for people who are not very active. This is an unfortunate reading of their true nature. Modern cardiac rehab is about pushing people to their full potential, and where possible, getting them even better than before, going back to work, or where they want to be – with controlled and methodical progress.

Exercise is essential into the years beyond rehabilitation as it is beneficial in managing risk factors and is crucial psychologically. The psychological health of a person after a heart event is a significant determinant of how well the person will do in the long term. Many studies show that regular exercise is as effective for improving mood as first-line antidepressant agents. So, as part of the rehabilitation process, finding physical activities that the person enjoys and will continue long-term is critical.

IMPORTANT POINTS

- Healing depends on
  - the invasiveness of the procedure undertaken,
  - the person's general health, and
  - the person's general fitness.
- Physical activity that is
  - progressively increased,
  - structured, and
  - supervised

  is the best approach to starting, or returning to, exercise.
- An exercise program needs to be tailored for the individual based on the person's needs rather than predetermined parameters and should include
  - aerobic activity, and
  - muscle strengthening.
- Exercise should be ongoing after rehabilitation for continued heart and other health benefits.

---

76 *The Institute of Advance Reconstruction, Dr Michael Rose MD FACS https://www.advancedreconstruction.com/pain-clicking-popping-chest-bone-heart-surgery/*

77 *https://www.heartfoundation.org.au/heart-health-education/physical-activity-and-exercise*
This reference also includes exercise recommendations for other age groups.
The World Health Organisation updated its guidelines on physical activity and sedentary behaviour in November 2020. A downloadable publication is available at https://www.who.int/publications/i/item/9789240015128 or a factsheet at https://www.who.int/news-room/fact-sheets/detail/physical-activity

78 *Weight training does not need to be heavy. Light to moderate intensity training resistance training is beneficial for recovery and long-term health and does not put the heart under undue stress.*

Cardiac recovery is more than a painful, physical journey. The emotions and one's mental stability also take a battering. If someone tells you that you are being grumpy, you probably are!

chapter 14
WHEN THE HEART GETS HEAVY

INTERVIEW ♥

Sense of self

Dr Bishop speaks with Ralf Ilchef

the Director of Liaison Psychiatry at Royal North Shore Hospital, Sydney, Australia.

WB I'm so pleased to have the opportunity to pick your brains about the process of recovering from a cardiac event because I think that mental side is just so important. As a liaison psychiatrist, you must come across people who have just had an event. What's your read with them, Ralf?

R *Psychiatrists think about it a bit differently to cardiologists. I work in a large teaching hospital and for anyone who doesn't know what a liaison psychiatrist is, it's a psychiatrist who sees people who have both medical and psychiatric problems. So, a large group of the people we see have been hospitalised for a cardiac event and are having some kind of issue with adjusting to it. That issue might be acute anxiety, or it might be low mood. Sometimes, it might be a pre-existing mental health problem that has been stirred up or worsened by a cardiac event.*

So, as a non-cardiologist I come to it almost as cleanly as a patient. We don't think about hearts very much. They're just these pumps that kind of work in our chest and then suddenly, something happens, and they stop working, or they stop working properly, and you get this terrible shock to your system.

There's a very profound sense of your own mortality. You're in the hands of these medical and health professionals. And you've got to try and make sense of this extraordinary thing that's happened to you.

We know that it's very, very common for people to have acute, what are called, 'adjustment reactions', anxiety or mood problems, collectively known as 'cardiac blues'. They happen very commonly. For most people, those things are brief, self-correcting and don't need any intervention. But about 20 per cent of people develop more significant mental health problems because of a cardiac event. Often this can be depression or an anxiety disorder. Some people can even have some elements of post-traumatic stress disorder (PTSD) because the threat to their life has been so profound. We get involved with those people of course.

But I think it's a massive event for anyone and I'm surprised by how well and how flexibly and adaptively and humorously the great majority of people react to these events.

WB When I see people after a heart event, I wonder if they're going through some sort of grieving process? The loss of good health, the loss of well-being, the loss of immortality being the things that they grieve. I can't remember the stages of the grieving process but there's anger and 'why me' and denial and so forth. Can you speak to that?

R *I think that what you have said is exactly right. There's nothing like an event happening to your heart to remind you that one day it is going to stop. That's a very profound recognition of your own mortality, and that's not something that people think about unless they're required to or made to. So, a cardiac event, I think, almost always has a huge impact on a person.*

The majority of people have an acute reaction. They deal with it well with the support of the health professionals they are working with and their families; they recover well and get on with their lives.

A significant group of people have these 'adjustment reactions', which are a little bit more than that. They are knocked out of orbit a bit longer by marked anxiety or by low mood – either worry or sadness, essentially – that are a bit more intense and a bit more prolonged and a bit more debilitating than usual. Most of those people don't need specific psychiatric help; they might need to see a psychologist or a counsellor or talk to their GP. ***For most of those people, in fact, engagement in a well-run and well-thought-out cardiac rehab program is probably the very best thing that you can do for them.***

And then you get this other group of people who have a more marked amount of debility associated with their cardiac event where they develop severe depression or severe anxiety or PTSD. Now, those people are really important to follow up because we know that, for example, untreated depression can affect the outlook after a cardiac event, increasing the impact that it has on a person's life. And it's not as simple as giving them an antidepressant or some counselling. They need a thoughtful and holistic approach to their rehabilitation to ensure that they have good outcomes.

WB Ralf, when people have a particularly rough road after their event, are there markers that are apparent before the event that we, as cardiologists, should be aware of? Is there a premorbid character who's going to have more troubles, or is it quite variable? Is it related to the extent of the injury or the event, say a heart attack versus a chest pain versus a cardiac arrest? What are your thoughts on that?

R *It's a great question and in fact, you know, some people are now saying that people who have a booked cardiac procedure should have some form of prehab; that they should really be looked at in terms of their risk factors* ***prior*** *to the cardiac surgery or the cardiac procedure because there are some things we know that put people at greater risk.*

The most obvious one, of course, is having had a past history of depression or a past history of an anxiety disorder or people who are known to have another mental health condition or, for example, an alcohol-use disorder or substance-use disorder. So, if a person has a history of mental health issues, then that person is definitely at increased risk after a cardiac event.

There used to be a lot said about personality types but that hasn't been well borne out in the literature and I think it can be misleading. However, there are certain things we also know put people at risk. People who have had more adversity, more struggles, in their life are more likely to have problems. As I have said, people with a history of depression or anxiety have problems.

Then, after that, it's a lot to do with the event itself:

- *how severe it was,*
- *how grave the threat to their sense of self was,*
- *how prolonged the hospital stay was,*
- *what they've been told about their prognosis, and*
- *how smooth or complicated their recovery was.*

All of these factors will have a big impact.

WB An observation from the clinical exposure I've had over more than 20 years of dealing with people in this space is that I get the sense that women deal with these challenges, or these events out of the blue, differently to men. I'm not sure who does better or worse, but I have the sense there is a difference. What are your thoughts?

R *(Although there is not much literature available on this topic) it is certainly possible that men and women react differently. We know that generally, for example, over a lifetime, women are more likely to experience depression than men, and more likely to experience anxiety. Men are more likely to experience substance-use disorders. So, there are certain mental health conditions that are more common in either men or women.*

I think it's also true that the health system treats men and women a bit differently, too.

Historically, we haven't been quite as good at picking cardiac problems in women as in men. It's known, for example, that the sort of chest pain that women get is often not quite as textbook as what we've been taught to understand is the chest pain of coronary artery disease. Other considerations can make their treatment in hospital a bit more complicated than men. So, it might be them responding to system issues, as opposed to vulnerability factors.

Off the top of my head, I don't know whether the rates of depression or anxiety are higher in women than in men. I don't imagine that there's an enormous difference because I've certainly seen plenty of people of both sexes who've suffered with depression and anxiety after cardiac events.

And of course, the symbolic impact of a loss of role to people is important too. Again, historically, men have tended to be a lot more invested in their work. That's obviously different now. Having to stop work or adjust your work can have a big psychological impact. Now that so many women also have busy careers that is less of a distinction.

WB One of the issues that's clearly different between the sexes is a potential loss of sexual function after an event. In my practice, it's not uncommon for men to report some loss of sexual function, at least for a time after an event. This is understandable for several reasons. There are the drugs, which can impact sexual function, but there must also be a fear of an event potentially occurring at any time and that must play on a person's mind. Do you deal with patients in that space and presumably there's a difference for men and women?

R *Absolutely. I've seen concerns expressed by both sexes, but probably the ones that come to mind most have been males who have been worried about resuming sexual function because of their concerns that it might trigger another cardiac episode and, also, because of problems with sexual function, either with arousal or in the case of men with achieving an erection or ejaculating. As you say, that can be for all sorts of factors including cardiac medications.*

And, of course, for people who are on medications for their mental health, anti-depressants can also have an impact on sexual function.

So, there are lots of reasons why it can be a bit of a minefield for people in the rehab period. It's an important part of recovering a healthy and full life and probably something that isn't as fully followed up and monitored as it should be.

WB It's a very important issue and I think it is often skirted around and pushed to one side.

One of the other things that I have observed is the importance of having a solid and supportive 'important other' in your life, your partner. There must be times when the partner is stressed or strained, or the partner may unravel. The benefit of having a strong partner is the support that that person can offer. Would you like to talk about partner, family, kids, and maybe even siblings? One of my areas of interest is prevention, and if Mr John Smith at 55 years of age has a heart attack, that's pretty young. So, the first thing I'd be asking is, have you got brothers or sisters?

R *Absolutely, Warrick. You've touched on so many things there.*

The amount of support that a person has is a vital determinant of the psychological recovery after a cardiac event.

For those who have a partner, for that person to be supportive and encouraging is really important. For those who don't, then certainly the roles of close friends, sibs, children, parents are significant. It's not something you want to be going through as an isolated person; you really need to have people on your side.

And of course, there is the couple relationship. A profound reorganisation of the dynamics of a relationship is needed because a person who has been an equal partner suddenly becomes acutely unwell and is now in this patient role, in this sick or invalid roll. A lot of things need to be renegotiated during that recovery period – and then as the patient recovers strength, those things need to be renegotiated back again. The partner who has been used to calling the shots for a while might not be that enthused about handing things back. So, there's a lot to work through. And, of course, as you mentioned earlier, the resumption of intimacy is a significant part of that period. So, for a couple there's plenty of areas to go through.

We know that attending a cardiac rehab program is important for recovery, *although a lot of people don't proceed or persist or complete these courses. There are all sorts of reasons: they want to get back to work, or they just don't want to think about it, or they hate being reminded that they've had an event.* ***A partner who is strongly encouraging of the need to complete the cardiac rehabilitation is a vital asset.***

WB I've done some reading around the advantage of having a positive partner and there's no question that individuals in stable, supportive relationships recover better.

R *It's certainly a great test for a relationship with everything being turned on its head and everything being made uncertain. Financial and every other sort of stress suddenly come into view, and so you get a sense of the mettle you're made of and what your partner is made of at a time like this.*

WB Another thing that I've observed is a difference in the response based on the age of the person. There's far more pragmatism and awareness of the transitory nature of life in our older patients who suffer events. They just seem more phlegmatic about it, which I guess is understandable. The younger ones are far more concerned, which I guess also makes sense. Do you see that?

R *I think that's right. You are constructing this narrative of your life as you go along.*

If you're a 75-year-old guy who's had a heart attack, and recovered from it, you get, well that's kind of something that happens at my time of life.

If you're a 35-year-old guy who has a heart attack, that's a very different story: Most of my mates, you know, are playing indoor cricket, or riding bikes, or going surfing and here I am holed up in a cardiac ward. *This sense of incredibly premature mortality is very frightening.*

So, psychologically, it's a much greater event for younger people, in their 30s, 40s, 50s, and that's definitely a predictor. I see those people as being at particular risk and needing the most intensive psychosocial and physical rehabilitation that we can offer them because I think that they're at higher risk of depression.

In this horrible circular movement, developing depression then worsens the outcome of the cardiac condition. And that's more complicated than it sounds because if a person who's had a cardiac event gets depression, unlike most people, you can't give them an antidepressant or send them off for six sessions of cognitive behavioural therapy, because that, by itself, is not very helpful as it doesn't improve the cardiac outcome. You've got to treat the depression, absolutely, but it's got to be locked in with every other phase of their risk reduction, and improving their fitness and improving their diet, and losing weight, and doing all the things that are required as part of their cardiac rehab.

And, certainly for the younger people, under 60s or so, I think they need more resources put into their treatment. An awful lot of cardiac rehab programs still don't have a strong psychological or psychosocial component to them. I think that's definitely an area for improvement.

WB Look, one of the things I find myself involved in with patients is trying to get them to take their tablets. "Take your medicine", I say, "it's good for you." And they say, "How long do I take it for, Doc?" And I say "For life. And that's a double meaning, so please take it!"

Compliance issues, Ralf. Do you think that people who have had bypass, a major procedure with a big scar and aches and pains, are psychologically better prepped because they've been greater impacted than someone who's wafted in with a bit of chest pain, gets a stent, goes back to work a week or two later, with barely a hair out of place, maybe a puncture site in the wrist or the leg? Tell me about your thoughts on compliance and taking medicine.

R *Medication adherence is a real problem, and the best thing for it is the quality of the therapeutic relationship they have, initially with their cardiologist and subsequently with their GP. Never underestimate the importance of explaining to them exactly what the drugs do and exactly why they're so important.*

We're not just saying this to fill up the consultation time, and because we've got nothing else to do, or because we want this drug company to take us away to a conference. We want you to take this pill, because there's really, really good evidence that it will improve your outcome.

Pushback from the patient is a good reminder to us to ask: Is this medication regimen as clean and efficient as it can be for this person? Are there any pills that we can stop? *As you know, doctors are fantastic at prescribing medication and we're terrible at stopping prescribing medications. Patients accrue medications like barnacles over time. So, every now and then, someone's got to look at them and say,* Do you still need to be on that blood pressure drug? When did we check your blood pressure? *I think you've got to be satisfied in your own mind that there's a powerful indication for them to be on that medication and then you've got to persuade them to stay on it. But adherence is a big issue, and, obviously, significant.*

WB Do you think the more profound nature of having your chest literally cracked open for a bypass focuses people's attention?

R *Oh, yeah. Nothing like a thoracotomy scar to remind you that this is real.*

WB There's no question of the value of rehabilitation, emotionally, and physically, as part of the process of recovering. Are you aware of any potential pitfalls or traps within the rehab process? I've observed some patients who go along and they compare number of grafts, for example.

R *I think like in every therapeutic group, there's always a risk that it will develop an unhealthy dynamic, captured by some large personality who has his or her own ideas. I think groups must be really well run and really well facilitated. Participants need to be reminded that everyone's story is different and that it's not actually relevant whether that one person had four grafts and another person had two, but that there are lots of other really important factors here. So, I think you are right.*

From my point of view, one of the great advantages of a rehab program is that at least those people are being seen and reviewed by skilled health clinicians on a regular basis. *They will notice if people are not coming to sessions, or if they're not saying very much. There are predictors of a possible bad outcome, such as,*

- *people with persistent physical symptoms that don't settle down;*
- *people with an unexpected reduction in exercise tolerance that isn't accounted for;*
- *people, while coming to sessions, seem very detached or whose mood deteriorates.*

It's great to have a rehab program so that those people get 'picked up', and then, hopefully, will at least talk to their GP about some follow-up that gets them the psychological and psychosocial support that they need.

Of course, there are risks whenever you get a group of people together, and people do get competitive, but ***overall, the rehab process is a really good one.***

WB Are there any signposts, or flags, for which an individual who has gone through a cardiac event, or the loved one, should be keeping an eye out? Something that would be the trigger for them to follow up with their GP?

R *Probably the loved one, especially because that person is the one who knows that the patient. It might be the patient's partner, close friend, parent or child, or whoever sees the person the most. There are a few things of which to be aware.*

Medication non-adherence is often a sign that a person is disengaged from the process and getting a bit fatalistic about things. That can be a sign of depression. Symptoms of depression that people ought to be aware of occur in three clusters.

*There are the **emotional** symptoms, like*

- *sadness*
- *teariness*
- *social withdrawal*
- *a sense of a foreshortened future*
- *a feeling of pessimism and hopelessness about everything.*

*There are also **physical** symptoms that can be quite hard to tease out from the physical symptoms that people who have just had a big cardiac procedure go through. These include*

- *fatigue*
- *loss of appetite*
- *sleep disturbance*
- *loss of sexual interest*
- *loss of pleasure in ordinarily pleasurable activities.*

*Then, there are also **cognitive** symptoms. It's not uncommon for people to have problems with memory and concentration and thinking after a big cardiac event. But, for people who find that their memory doesn't work very well, that they can't plan very well, it can also be a hint that the depression is an issue.*

Lapsing into behaviours that are obviously not good for them like

- *resuming a bad diet*
- *resuming smoking*
- *drinking too much*
- *passive-aggressively defying all the medical advice that they've been given,*

is often a sign that a person is demoralised and getting quite depressed. This becomes an opportunity for an intervention to turn it around. A patient's GP is a great place to start.

WB We've covered an enormous amount of ground. I've learned so much from you. Is there anything with which you'd like to close? Maybe you have a parting remark on something that you really want to underline? This is an extraordinary, extraordinary moment in people's lives – and an opportunity for us to think about it and do it better. You've focused me to pay more attention in that space, no question.

R *There's nothing like a major cardiac event to make people have a reset in their life and to do what they can do to resume control of their life, improve their physical health, improve their relationships. Think about the impact of depression and anxiety. We've talked so far about heart disease predisposing people to depression, but it's important to know that depression predisposes you to heart disease. So, people living with depression are putting themselves at risk. Mental health is always something that you want to optimise as much as you can. So, it's a great opportunity to really give yourself a 20,000-kilometre service and have your mental and emotional health seen to along with your physical health.*

And remember, there's never been a better time to have a cardiac event. Medicine has come such a long way. There are so many wonderful treatments available, and more coming down the tube, so that people should feel confident that they've never been better placed to have a good outcome from a cardiac event – to be confident that they have a lot of life ahead of them and that they should live it as well as they can.

WB I'm going to end with a plug for an area of rehab that I think is incredibly important. That is the role of exercise, for not only things like blood pressure, strength, mobility, sugar control, insulin resistance, but it's also good for mood and, correct me if I'm wrong, exercise can be as effective as an antidepressant.

R *That's absolutely correct, Warrick, and, in fact, the news is all good. Any amount of moderately vigorous physical activity that you do is good for mood and anxiety. The great news is it doesn't matter what the exercise is. If you like weightlifting, that's fine. If you like running, that's fine. If you like playing golf, that's fine. Anything that gets you out and gets your heart rate up is really good for mood and really good for anxiety. The optimal amount is about an hour a day or seven hours a week.*

Plenty of people can't do that much and that's fine. Any more than that, you're very welcome to do if you enjoy it, but that doesn't confer any additional mood or anxiety benefit on you. Regular physical activity is a fantastic thing to incorporate into your life, purely from a mood and anxiety perspective.

from the Darren Lehmann interview

You read earlier that Darren said that recovery was a tough process, mentally ... *(initially) you're scared because you could leave them behind. You're going into open-heart surgery, but what if it goes wrong? You just don't know, do you?*

DARREN continues *(further into the recovery) I suppose the biggest one for me has been the mental side of it. I have good days and bad days, and that's no secret. There are days when I just don't feel like doing anything or I just feel like sitting outside and smelling the fresh air, which is something I didn't know if I would do again or not.*

You have good days and bad days. You just have to have people around you who you can talk to about what you're feeling. It is so important. You wake up and you feel, I'm up and I'm ready to go again, *but then you feel flat and ask* Why's this happened to me?

Later, you look back on your journey and you understand why. You can't look back at that stage.

What's happened is in the past, and I cannot worry about that. I've got to worry about things that are important – my family, obviously, and into the future, and living life to the fullest as long as I possibly can. As the doctor said, You know, we just put a V8 engine back in you. Make sure you look after it this time.

That's the hardest thing. I might be sitting quietly at home. And, you know, I do things I've never done before. Now I read a lot more. I listen to podcasts and music. And if I don't want to do something, I just don't do it now. I just say, No. I don't really want to do that, thank you. I'm not doing it.

You don't have so much politics in your brain. You simplify things, because everything brings it back to a really simple view – that your family are the most important thing in your life. We worry about everyone else when we really should be just looking within and really concentrating on the important ones.

When you go through this whole process, you get a lot of good messages and messages of support, and that's so important. I've been lucky to have a great support of family and friends who are very understanding.

interconnectedness

"(Cardiovascular disease - CVD) should not be addressed as an isolated entity but rather as one part of an integrated system in which mind, heart, and body are interconnected. Both positive psychological status and negative psychological status appear to affect cardiovascular health and prognosis directly. Wellness and well-being involve not only physical factors but also psychological ones. Clinicians should strive to treat not just the disease state but the patient and the person as a whole."

This is the concluding paragraph of a statement by the American Heart Association issued in January 2021.[79] The statement's conclusions[80] are:

- Psychological health is an important component of wellness/well-being for patients with or at risk for CVD.
- The mind, heart, and body are all interconnected and interdependent in a relationship that can be called the mind-heart-body connection.
- There is a substantial body of good-quality data showing clear associations between psychological health and CVD and risk.
- There is increasing evidence that psychological health may be causally linked to biological processes and behaviors that contribute to and cause CVD.
- The preponderance of data suggest that interventions to improve psychological health can have a beneficial impact on cardiovascular health. Simple screening measures can be used by health care clinicians for patients with or at risk for CVD to assess psychological health status.
- Consideration of psychological health is advisable in the evaluation and management of patients with or at risk for CVD.

IMPORTANT POINTS

- Be kind to yourself.
- Let those around you be kind to you.
- Be aware of the interconnectedness of body, mind and heart.

---

79 *Psychological Health, Well-Being, and the Mind-Heart-Body Connection: A Scientific Statement from the American Heart Association; originally published 25 Jan 2021 https://doi.org/10.1161/CIR.0000000000000947 Circulation. 2021;143:e763–e783*

80 *ibid.*

Resuming 'normal' life.

chapter 15

WHEN CAN I . . . ?

As you recover from your cardiac trauma – be it an event or a diagnosis – you begin to look to resume 'normal life'. Often, though, activities that used to be 'normal' are now shrouded in uncertainty and wariness.

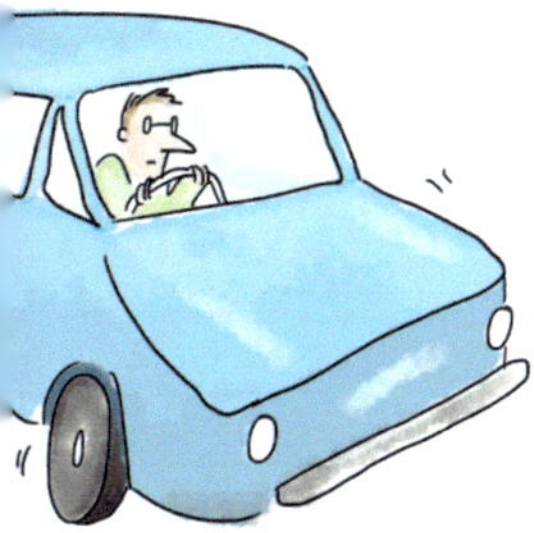

drive

In most instances, a person can drive after suffering a heart event. However, guidelines need to be followed and these depend on the country in which the person lives and sometimes the requirements of even more local jurisdictions.

Distinctions are also made between private and commercial use licenses.

The length of time between the event and a return to driving ranges from 24 hours to months depending on the heart event suffered. In several specific instances, a return to commercial driving is not allowed.

From a cardiac perspective, one of the main determinants is the limitation in chest movement, governed by how much trauma the chest suffers because of the cardiac event. Inserting a pacemaker or a stent is minor surgery. Bypass grafting is major surgery that has a significant impact on the chest, so that not only is there internal repair around the heart, the chest itself also needs to heal.

It is important that when in a car, either as the driver or passenger, that the seat belt be worn, and remember to follow the Transport Commission Guidelines, or those of your local authority, for resumption of driving.

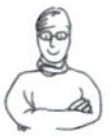

It would be a shame to save someone from a heart attack only to have the person die in a car accident from not wearing a seatbelt.

in broad terms[81]	private	commercial
blackout	• a simple faint might be 24 hours • is it a cardiac problem, neurological, or brain related? • if a cause is found, can it be fixed? • will the problem reoccur?	a simple faint might be 24 hours with the licensing authority notified any other cause, a three-month non-driving period, subject to specialist review
heart attack	2 weeks	4 weeks
pacemaker	2 weeks	4 weeks
stent	2 days	4 weeks
bypass graft	4 weeks	3 months
cardiac arrest	6 months	6 months
implant of cardioverter defibrillator	6 months after cardiac arrest	not applicable

A commercial driver's license requires additional clearance precautions to the above considerations. Generally, further testing is mandated in the guidelines, including an ultrasound (echo) and functional testing. The echo assesses the pumping capacity of the heart and provides a figure called the ejection fraction. This needs to be close to normal to qualify a person for a commercial vehicle license. The functional test, often using a treadmill, also provides information that helps determine if a person is safe to return to driving a commercial vehicle. A conditional licence can be considered subject to annual review by a cardiologist.

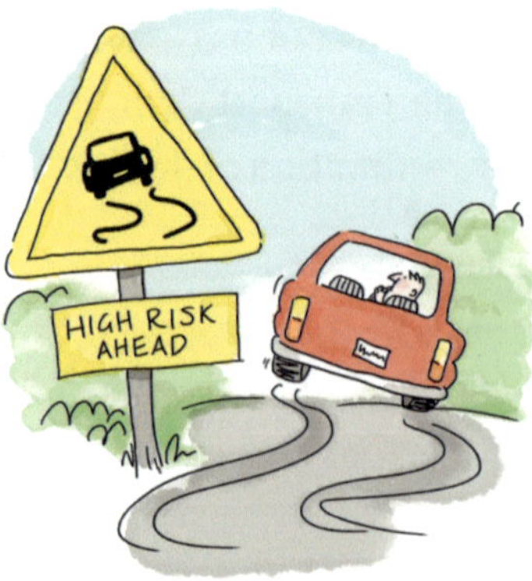

For either form of licence, failure to follow the guidelines may have outcomes, such as insurance not covering liability.

While driving is a huge form of independence for most people of all ages, it is not a right. Safety for the person and other road users is paramount. As there are many nuances with each individual, on-going discussions with the cardiologist are vital.

exercise

A structured cardiac rehabilitation program is the best way to begin exercising after a cardiac event or diagnosis. Your fitness level can be assessed by professionals and matched with your cardiac recovery/ health. Your progress can be monitored, and you will receive support and encouragement. *(for more information on exercise, please refer to chapters 13 and 18)*

have sex

Questions related to having sex are common. The bottom line is, it depends on the severity of your heart condition and limitations to your exercise capacity. Technically, there is no restriction to you being physically active sexually if you have had a cardiac problem. In reality, though, you need physical energy to have sex. If you can climb, say, three flights of stairs, and not be short of breath, or are able to undertake some light exercise, you should have the exercise capacity required for sexual intimacy.

Some cardiac medications can lead to erectile dysfunction. Drugs, such as spironolactone, thiazides, and beta-blockers have been known to dampen sexual function.

This leads to the question, *Can I use Viagra?* Generally, the Viagra-type, phosphodiesterase inhibitor drugs can be used. However, there is a **cautionary note.** If coronary artery disease (narrowed arteries) is the cause of your heart problem, then be very careful to check you are not taking nitrate-based medication which includes the spray under the tongue. These medications dilate blood vessels to help the arteries. They react with Viagra and can drop the blood pressure profoundly and dangerously. It is wise to have a conversation with your cardiologist or your local doctor.

work

This one will be determined by the job and your ability to physically perform the required tasks. Apart from the driving-related restrictions discussed above, there remains a very real and practical issue which is, *Are you able to perform your required duties for work safely and effectively?*

Large organisations most likely will have return-to-work processes in place, while smaller organisations may require a 'clearance' from your cardiologist or your local doctor or maybe a rehabilitation physician.

Generally, your cardiologist will be a good starting point for the journey back to work and, of course, valued input can be obtained from the experienced cardiac rehab team who will know you well from your rehab experience.

travel

The simple answer to the question, *Can I travel?* is, *Yes, possibly*. The "possibly" means that you need to be aware of

- your own recovery
- your own limitations and, of course,
- the travelling conditions and destination.

As the amount of activity required will be important, it would be sensible to have a good idea before you go of what will be expected from you physically. Perhaps, even check with your cardiologist if a stress test would help inform your decision-making.

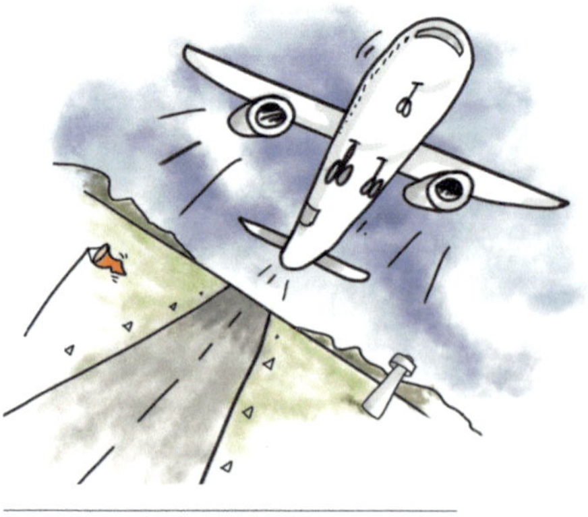

Even for people without cardiac failure, long flights are hard work.

If you have heart failure and you are planning to travel by air, the effect of decompression in the cabin, to an altitude of between 8000 and 10,000 feet, needs to be considered.

For patients whose condition is unstable, air travel is not a good idea. Less oxygen than you are used to at sea level could destabilise or worsen your condition.

Generally, however, that change in oxygenation should not be a problem on short trips for patients who are taking their medications, have been recently reviewed, and whose condition has stabilised and is well maintained.

Longer trips present complications.

The timing of medications is important, both on the ground and in the air. Fluid tablets, for example, can pose challenges. Dehydration can easily occur on a long-haul flight, or you might become cramped and through lack of mobility, run the risk of clots forming in the legs. So, consideration of long-haul flights is something that needs a thoughtful approach.

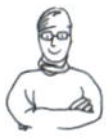

Remember, flying commercially is not permitted within 10 days of open-heart surgery. Beyond that, your future travel plans would make a great conversation with your cardiologist.

As a traveller, you also need to think about your arrival destination. Flying to a high-altitude destination could precipitate problems because of change in oxygenation. Flying from sea level directly to a high-altitude destination such as Las Pas, in Bolivia, could cause headache and early signs of altitude sickness even in the 'fit' population. **Be aware**, if you have heart issues, acute decompensation and, certainly, decreased exercise capacity, could be your first memory of your high-altitude holiday.

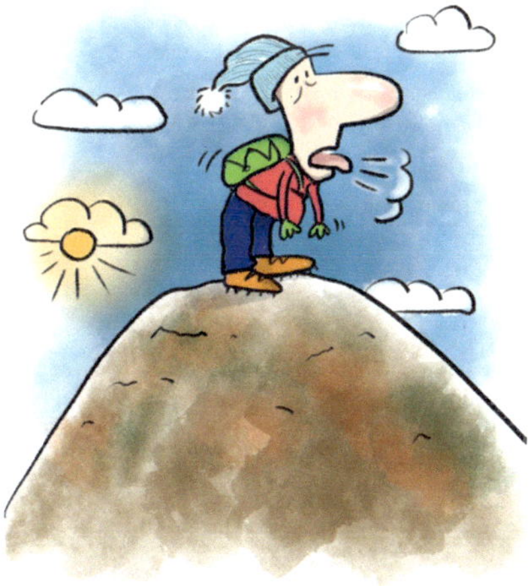

If you have cardiac failure, doing the Annapurna Circuit or an Everest Base camp trek should probably not be on your bucket list.

have vaccinations

Vaccinations are vital - particularly in this COVID world.

With cardiac issues, you are at increased risk of contracting multiple, different conditions. Work with your doctor to ensure that you are appropriately vaccinated.

Recent inflammation of the sac around your heart (the pericardium), or recent inflammation of the heart muscle (myocarditis), could be a reason to hold off on vaccination for COVID pending specialist advise.

In general terms, however, heart problems related to rhythm, valves or the blood vessels (coronary artery disease) should not prevent vaccination.

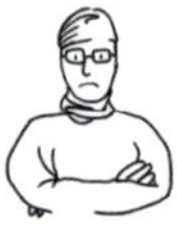

NO QUESTION! NO ARGUMENT!
Pneumococcal, flu and COVID vaccines are highly recommended if you have impaired heart function.

IMPORTANT POINTS

- **driving**
  - most people can drive after a heart event, although local guidelines need to be followed. Distinctions are made between private and commercial licences.
  - a significant cardiological factor is the chest movement, determined by how much trauma the chest has suffered. Don't start using a car, particularly as driver, too early.
- **exercising**
  - a structured rehabilitation program under the watchful eye of a professional is the best way to begin (and possibly continue).
- **sex**
  - how severe is your heart condition?
  - how good is your exercise capacity?
  - take special care with drug interactions if you are using Viagra-type medications.
- **work**
  - are you able to perform your required duties for work safely and effectively?
- **travel**
  - yes – possibly, if you are aware of
    - > your recovery
    - > your limitations
    - > the nature of your travelling conditions and your destinations.
  - be prepared if using either domestic or international flights.
- **vaccinations**
  - **yes!**

81 *in Australia, based on the national guidelines from the National Transport Commission*

There is life after a cardiac event. A near-death experience brings a new passion into the life of Greg Page, a passion that has the potential to save many lives.

chapter 16

LIFE AFTER A CARDIAC EVENT

INTERVIEW ♥

Beating the odds

Dr Bishop speaks with Greg Page AM[82]

an Australian singer, musician, and actor who was a founding member, the lead singer and the original Yellow Wiggle in the internationally successful phenomenon, The Wiggles, an Australian children's entertainment band.

The precipitating event was an Original Wiggles[83], adults-only, concert held in January 2020 to raise funds for victims of the devastating bushfires of the 2019-2020 Australian summer. Greg Page 'died' on stage at the end of the concert.

WB ... I'm going to ask just a little bit about yourself. How old are you and what's your family background about heart disease? We're not going to talk too much about The Wiggles today.

G *No problem. Much more important things to focus on today. So, I'm now 48-years-old. And there's no real family history of heart disease. My grandmother did have high cholesterol. She lived until she was in her late 80s. And she did have a heart attack at 68 and had a subsequent heart attack and then a stroke. So yes, she did have some heart disease, but it's not like everybody in my family has some form of heart disease triggers.*

So, it's an interesting thing when doctors ask you, What's your family history? *And if you don't know it, it's very hard to answer correctly. So, I guess this is what makes it difficult for doctors to be able to kind of diagnose your risk of heart disease if you don't know your family history very well.*

WB It's true.

What about other things, Greg? You are 48 years of age. You're not overweight; we know that. Were you exercising regularly? Did you look after your diet? Were you someone who thought you were doing all the right things or were there things, looking back now, that suggest you weren't looking after yourself as well as you might have been?

G *A bit of both. About 13 or 14 years ago, I was quite heavy. I think I was probably about 109 kilos, which was too much. So, towards the end of my time with The Wiggles, I'd put on a bit of weight. We had trainers and people coming on board to ensure we were as fit as possible because The Wiggles' shows were quite physically demanding. To make sure we were doing the best we could we had nutritionists and dietitians consult and give advice.*

I'm not a good eater. I'm a very fussy eater, and that goes back to my childhood. I don't eat a lot of fruit and veg. I eat a lot of meat; I used to eat a lot of probably fatty meat, to be honest. Then, that turned around for me about 13 years ago when I met my wife, Vanessa. She's a cardiac nurse. She looked at my diet, she looked at my weight, and she tried to get me to change. I changed, but in retrospect, I probably didn't change enough.

I exercised a lot. I always enjoy exercising. I like being what I call 'fit' but being fit isn't the same as being healthy. And that's what I now know. So, I thought, Okay, my diet is not the best, but I'm exercising: I walk, I play cricket, I play tennis, I go to the gym, I work out. I can do all of that without getting the typical symptoms of, "Gosh, I've got a heavy chest" *or you know,* "I feel unwell"*, those kinds of things. So, I think it's a little bit of both. I look back now and think,* You know, I wasn't really looking after myself as well as I should have been.

WB Those lifestyle considerations are important. But did you have the benefit of knowing what your cholesterol measurements were, or blood pressure? The other thing, of course, is I'm guessing you've never smoked?

G *No. Look, I've had a few cigarettes, trying to be cool, you know, back in the day, but I was never a habitual smoker, and .... I never inhaled either.*

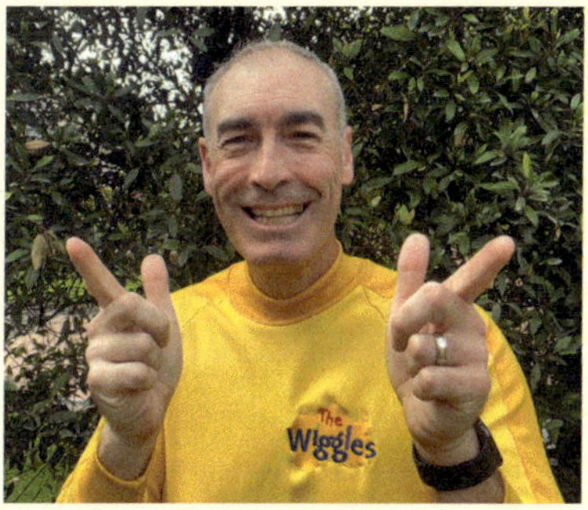

WB Cholesterol and blood pressure? Were you aware of them? Were they a problem?

G *Going back about maybe seven or eight years ago, my cholesterol reading was 6.2. That, again, was a signal to change my diet. I changed my diet and I did introduce a lot more salad. Like, I never used to eat salad! Then, Vanessa came along, and she got me eating salad at least. I kind of thought changes like that were enough because I was exercising. It's not as if my diet was absolutely abominable. I wasn't eating, you know, fast food takeaway every night of the week, greasy hamburgers or greasy, oily chicken. I'd have some of those things every now and then but I wasn't gorging on those kinds of foods. So, I thought,* Okay, well, I'm having some of that every now and then. I'm having the food that I enjoy, which wasn't unhealthy, *I didn't think. Looking back, I probably had too much cheese in my diet. I probably had too much pizza, toasted ham and cheese sandwiches or lasagne with cheese on top. Those kinds of things.*

WB You sound very much like an average 40-something-year-old bloke who'd put on a bit of weight then lost a bit of weight. Maybe could have eaten a bit better, but you did a bit of exercise. You didn't have much in the way of a family history as a flag. Your cholesterol was a bit on the high side, but not catastrophically high. From what you described, there's no major flag, Greg, and that really leads us on to the guts of this interview, which is the event that you had. I heard it on the news, as I guess many people did. Can you walk me through what happened? Was it last year?

G *There's not a lot I can remember to be honest.*

So, the 17th of January was the day after my 48th birthday. We had this performance to do for The Wiggles. I was very conscious that I had to do a show; we hadn't done a show in some time. So, I was conscious about my physical fitness. I'd been walking and exercising, staying relatively fit. I don't remember a lot about the day itself, nor the show… But one of the things I can remember is lying on the ground after I'd collapsed – you know, going into cardiac arrest.

With the benefit of hindsight, I can tell everybody that what happened physiologically inside my body ***was a clot had formed in my LAD, my left anterior descending artery, in my heart and blocked off that artery. Apparently 100 per cent. And almost immediately, I would say, I went into cardiac arrest.***

I don't remember any warning signs. I don't remember feeling heavy in the chest or any pain or any shortness of breath, other than what I would normally experience during a Wiggles' show when you're being physically active and exerting yourself. I was out of breath, and that's what I can remember. I don't remember the moment of collapsing, but I do remember lying on the floor, looking up at the ceiling, and struggling to breathe. I remember thinking, Gosh, I'm **so** out of breath. I'm **so** exhausted after that show, *but I didn't think that that could have been my last few breaths on this earth.*

WB Was that memory – of you lying on the floor looking up – after you had been resuscitated, Greg?

G *I think that was before I passed out. It was like, the last few breaths I was taking. Luckily, people around me recognised that I was in cardiac arrest or that I needed CPR (cardio-pulmonary resuscitation) and they jumped straight onto it. Called triple zero, of course, and then straight into the CPR. So, I'm very, very fortunate.*

WB Kerry Packer, who survived a cardiac arrest when he was playing polo, if you remember, many years ago, remarked that there was nothing on the other side. Did you have any awareness of something else? Do you recall anything from it?

G *No. The only thing I can recall are those last few breaths and just feeling really tired. Struggling to breathe, I guess. I felt like I was struggling to swallow. You know, when you get that lump in your throat and you're trying to swallow. I felt like I was trying to swallow and I couldn't.*

Look, apart from that, I didn't feel distress of any sort. I didn't know what was happening. And no, there was nothing on the other side, I think only because I didn't make it to the other side. Thank goodness, people got to me in time. If we want to talk in spiritual terms, I do believe there is something on the other side, but I don't believe I got there because of the actions of those people around me... I might have been technically dead because my heart wasn't beating for itself; it was in ventricular fibrillation[84]*. But I don't think I died. I nearly died, but I didn't actually die.*

WB Just to reiterate, and I think this is so important, from what you're describing, up until that moment – from your exercise, your day-to-day physical exertion – there was no clue that something might happen?

G *No. I'll tell you this, too. You asked earlier about cholesterol. About four or five weeks before this event, so back in December 2019, I'd been to my GP to get a blood test done for something else. I asked her to check my cholesterol because I hadn't had a check for a while.*

So, when the test came back, and cholesterol reading was 6.6, I asked her if it was anything to worry about? She said that as I hadn't fasted before the test, it was possibly not accurate and that I should watch what I was eating and keep doing my exercise.

So, I did that, and nothing kind of alarmed me... (After my admission to hospital) they did cholesterol the next morning, after I had fasted, and it was 4.8. So, I don't know. Even if I had had a proper cholesterol test done back in December, a month before my cardiac arrest, I don't know if it would have revealed anything when had I been fasting because I don't think a 4.8 overall cholesterol is that high to worry about, is it?

WB There are two things that come out of that. One is that cholesterol, of its own, in predicting who's going to have a problem, is not always accurate. It's very, very important once we know you've got a problem, because lowering it will make a difference, but it's not a great predictor.

The other thing that I think is really important, Greg, is you present as one of the individuals who has an event in an artery, where the artery, until the time the plaque ruptures, is not flow-limiting, not stopping blood getting down the artery. We know about 50 per cent of heart attacks occur on arteries that are not narrowed until the plaque ruptures and that clot forms. And I think that's the scary bit, isn't it?

G *It really is, because, as I said, I could exercise. I'd play cricket. You know, I remember in December I bowled 17 overs in a day. Now, for a 47-year-old, that's not bad – charging in, trying to bowl your fastest 17 overs in one afternoon. And I didn't feel like I was struggling.*

And a couple of weeks back, I met a woman who told me she was having a heart attack for six weeks before she got treated. She said she was having some uncomfortable feeling in her chest, and eventually she went and was seen. And she was told that she'd had a massive heart attack. Going back six weeks, they could tell that her heart was damaged. She said she'd lost a third of her heart function because of this massive heart attack over six weeks (from which) she wasn't really feeling symptoms.

So, I know that's not directly related to what we're talking about, but the point is, I think the symptoms of heart attack can be put down to other things. People aren't necessarily aware. So, for me, any shortness of breath that I might have been feeling I was putting down to the fact that I was exercising and I was just a little bit older now. So, I'd do my seven-and-half kilometre walk, I'd get back, and I think, Gee, that was a good walk. I'm pretty puffed after that. I was going pretty hard, so, you know, I'm probably justified in feeling the way I feel. *But what I can say now is, that after having a stent put in, I can do that same walk, and I can do it quicker than I did before and not be as puffed.*

So, I think for some people, perhaps, some of those little indicators are there, but we don't recognise them because we just think it's only that one thing. I'm not out of breath **and** feeling heavy in the chest, **and** I'm not getting pain in the neck or the jaw or the arm. *It's not **all** the warning signs that we get told to look for. It's maybe one of them and so we think,* Oh, well, look, I've got high cholesterol, I'll be fine, *or, you know,* I've got shortness of breath, but I'm getting older. *So, I don't know. I'm not the doctor.*

WB It can be incredibly subtle for something that hits you like a sledgehammer. And I think that's what your story is – subtle indicators and wham!

G *It's a very interesting series of events, I guess.*

Greg told Dr Bishop that his memory of following events was like kind of remembering it but without any solid memory. He said that it wasn't until he was in a ward the next morning, after the implantation of a stent, while speaking with a nurse that reality dawned. She told him that he had suffered a cardiac arrest and that his chest would be sore from when he had received CPR.

G *That's when it really hit me as to what had happened. I didn't still realise at that point the difference between a cardiac arrest and a heart attack, but I knew that if someone had been performing CPR on me, I must have been in a bad way. So that was my first kind of moment of acknowledgement of how serious that night was. And the next thing that really shocked me was hearing that I was the one in 10 who survive. Ten per cent of people survive a cardiac arrest. And then it really hit home, very hard.*

WB It's staggering.

During that time in hospital, what surprised you – doctors or nurses or procedures, ultrasounds on your heart, drips in? What are the things that really impacted you?

G *Okay. Nothing impacted me in a bad way or negative way. I think I was really overcome with gratefulness to be alive still, and you know, I had this second chance to look at my life again and do things differently. I realised that I almost didn't have that chance, that I almost wasn't there.*

The whole time in hospital is a blur still for me.

The important part of this is that what I do remember is getting up and about and being told that I've got to get into cardiac rehab. That was interesting for me because that started the whole process of **What is cardiac rehab? What do I have to do now to keep my heart functioning well going forward?**

And, so, I guess, one good thing was that ***cardiac rehab consisted mostly of walking****. You know, exercise, and getting the heart rate up to a certain level; not over-exerting but doing enough to make it work and keep it conditioned. I guess one thing they've learned over the years is that if you tell people after cardiac arrest to just lie in bed and don't do anything, the heart will become deconditioned perhaps, and it won't necessarily regain its ability to be as strong. I was glad to hear that walking was part of rehab because I love my walking and I was glad to be able to get back out and do that.*

WB Tell me, Greg, did rehab roll straight on from the end of your time in hospital? How long were you in hospital?

G *I was in hospital for five days and I think* ***I was home for about a week before I went to my first rehab session****. There, we touched a little bit on diet, and they explained to me what had happened within my heart, the physiology of the blockage and why I went into cardiac arrest. Then, it was pretty much just about weight checks, body density I think it would be called – you know, muscle mass versus fat mass – and then stress test and then,* Okay, here's your walking program. This is what you need to do to get that heart rate up. *It was really quite interesting.*

I was surprised how hard I had to walk to get my heart rate up to the level that they wanted. And that could have been because of the beta-blockers as they affect the ability of the heart to get up to the 130s, 140s. I think 133, 134 was where they wanted my heart rate. And I found that that was quite challenging. I thought, Wow! I'm having to work harder than I did before I had my cardiac arrest and, here I am, passing all these people on the walking track. I've just had a cardiac arrest and I'm overtaking them, trying to get my heart rate up.

WB For anyone who doesn't know what a beta-blocker is, it's a drug that dampens down the sympathetic nervous system, our 'fight or flight' nervous system, the one that makes your heart race and makes your legs ready to run or fight. So, beta-blockers reduce your heart rate, blood pressure and the risk of subsequent heart attack or cardiac arrest.

But tell me Greg, you obviously understand a little bit more about medicine now, and you're obviously taking a few medications. What's your understanding of these medications? Can you tell me what you're on? Do you carry a list, as I always ask my patients to? And can you explain what each medication is for?

G *Well, I think I can.*

In the morning, I have an anticoagulant tablet. I'll be on that one for probably the first year and that is to stop the chance of re-stenosis of the stent, to stop the blood clotting around the stent that's inside the artery. I'm on aspirin as well. That's a blood thinner to stop the chance of a blood clot generally happening and is not specifically to do with the stent. And I'll be on aspirin probably for the rest of my life.

WB Before you jump on to the next one, I'll explain a little bit further.

The aspirin and the other tablet both stop the stickiness of the small particles in the blood that can promote clot formation, generally, or a clot forming on the stent. And, so, aspirin, you'll be on for life because it'll stop clots forming in the arteries. And we're doubling it up for about a year, during the time the stent is most likely to be exposed to the contents of the blood. During that time, the lining of the blood vessel where the stent has been implanted, will grow over that stent. Then you can stop the second agent. So, these tablets work together. They are called dual anti-platelet (DAPT) agents.

G *Dual antiplatelet agents. There you go!*

WB They are blood thinners.

G *In the morning, I'm also on a smaller dose of the beta-blocker and a potassium tablet and two magnesium tablets. The beta-blocker is, as I said before, to give the heart a chance to rest so it doesn't get the rate up too high and also to prevent that chance of a potential follow up cardiac arrest. The potassium and the magnesium, I guess, are electrolytes. Is that how we would put it? Because having irregularities in your electrolytes can also lead to the chance of cardiac arrest in patients, too.*

WB Are you on a cholesterol tablet?

G *Yes. That's night-time. So, night-time is cholesterol and another beta-blocker, a higher dose of the beta-blocker at night-time, and more magnesium. That's it in terms of medications. There are a couple of other things I take as well, like Co-enzyme Q10 or CoQ10.*

WB Co-enzyme Q10 or CoQ10 or ubiquinone. That's a part of an enzymatic system which is involved with energy production throughout the body. There's some literature that suggests it's helpful for hearts and it can be beneficial for people who are on statins to reduce the risk of side-effects. It's a nice supplement. It's not supported by the PBS, but your local health food store or chemist will help you with it.

G *And the other one that I have is hawthorn.*

WB Blood pressure lowering.

G *Yeah, that's right. So that's pretty much my list of meds and my understanding of what they do.*

WB Good.

Now, the rehab program you went to, how long did that run, Greg?

G *That was six weeks. And I did what they call the home walking program. Rather than going every week to the rehab centre at the hospital, I did a home walking program for six weeks.*

On the first visit, they did a stress test, and there were no concerns. Then, at the end of the six weeks, we did another stress test. They put me on the treadmill, again, with the ECG, and there had been some improvements. *So – this is where I must remember what it was – I think there was a T wave inversion on my first ECG. Does that sound right, a T wave?* (WB, Yeah.) *So, that had corrected itself by the end of the six-week rehab. They were happy. There was no problem with my physical fitness in either of those stress tests.* ***So, I'm very, very fortunate that I was so fit, relatively, before I had my cardiac arrest. I think that played a big part in my ability to bounce back.***

Look, ***the worst part about it for me was the broken ribs for the six or seven weeks after the event from the CPR****. And I do remember having a kind of uncomfortable feeling in the chest for probably that six or seven weeks. I don't know, it might have hung on a little bit past that. I don't know whether that was my heart feeling a bit funny, but that's gone now. At the time, I just thought it was my ribs, but it's a different feeling. Like, I can remember what it felt like, so, I'm not too sure what that was. But it's all good, now.*

WB It can take about eight weeks for bones to heal. So, it can be a while. Normally, there's not too much left-over pain from the heart, per se. Very occasionally, the sac around the heart can become inflamed after a heart attack, and you can get a thing called pericarditis, a sharp and localised pain that changes with position. It doesn't sound like you had that.

G *I don't know what it was. Maybe it was just to do with the ribs. But that's all gone now. And I feel better than 100 per cent.*

WB Did they tell you if there was damage to your heart muscle, Greg?

G *Yes. So, the ejection fraction, is that what they call it?* (WB, Yes.) *LV EF, the left ventricle ejection fraction*[85]*?* (WB, Yes.) *Now, I'm going to try and remember the numbers here because I know it's gone back into the normal range. What's the bottom end of the normal range? Is it 45 per cent? ... Okay. Well, I think it was 45 per cent because they were umming and ahhing about whether or not to put in an ICD*[86]*, an internal defibrillator.* (WB, Yes.) *Because it was 45 and kind of borderline, they didn't want to worry about it. Then after all the rehab, the ejection fraction went back up. And gosh, as I said, I can't remember, but it's now back up into a more normal range. It might be 55 now, I think.*

WB That's in the normal range, which is great. It's good news for you. What about you, yourself? When did you start to feel more normal?

G *Pretty much straightaway. I was very fortunate.*

WB We've gone through your rehab, the event, and what led up to the event. Now, we are in the here and now. How has this impacted your life, Greg, because it's a big thing?

G *Yeah, look, it is a big thing. I view every day now as a bonus, and I have a mission. I'm still doing the other things that I used to do. That is, I'm still working in the children's entertainment field and trying to do what I can to produce shows for children.* ***But I'm now on a mission*** *to educate older people as well, about heart disease and cardiac arrest, and the difference between cardiac arrest and heart attack, and CPR (cardio-pulmonary resuscitation) and AED (automated external defibrillator)*[87]*.*

Given that stat about how many people survive a cardiac arrest and the fact that it is so low, I think we've got a long way to go in terms of educating people about response to cardiac arrest and improving those outcomes for people. So, ***more people knowing CPR, having more AEDs available and knowing where they are and how to use them*** *– there's a big mission there for me that I really feel compelled to be contributing towards.*

WB For those (reading) who are not up with the abbreviated terms, what are they, Greg?

G *CPR stands for cardio-pulmonary resuscitation, and AED stands for automated external defibrillator.*

And so, one of the big things about AEDs, or those defibrillators, that people probably don't understand, is that you don't need to be medically qualified or certified to use one to save a life. On the night that I needed to be shocked with an AED, there was a nurse there, but any one of those bystanders could have used that AED to shock my heart back into a normal rhythm. And that's what people need to know – you can't hurt somebody by using an AED because it will not shock somebody who doesn't need to be shocked. The pads that you place on the chest of the patient will determine if that patient needs to be shocked. And the AED talks to you and tells you what to do. It will only say push the shock button if it needs to deliver a shock to that patient. And you, as the user of the device, can't be harmed, either.

WB From a completely practical point of view, CPR and AED saved your life, Greg. That's the only reason we're talking.

G *Yep, absolutely. Because if you don't start CPR within the first, well, I've heard within the first three minutes, your brain will start to die because there's only enough oxygen within your blood to keep your organs oxygenated for around three minutes. So, if that blood isn't pumping around the body, then it's not going to keep things going. It's a critical process.*

An area of special interest for Dr Bishop is preventative cardiology – trying to stop people having an initial problem. He said that, in cardiology terms, Greg, as a 48-year-old male, would be seen as having premature coronary artery disease and someone whose family could be at high risk. He asked about Greg's siblings.

G *... I've spoken to my sister about it, but I don't know what she's done about it. She's having a birthday in a couple of weeks, so I better make sure that she sees a doctor before her birthday. If my track record is anything to go by, I don't want her to have her birthday and then have something go wrong the next day. I know she's on top of her health ... but in terms of cardio-vascular issues, I'm not sure.*

WB ... Looking at family members closes that loop of rehab in a sensible way. Just ask that question, so people don't get surprised.

So, a couple more questions. Have you noticed if your mood, relationships, interactions have been affected by this event? Are you back in your normal headspace, again?

G *Look, I'm not in the same headspace because, if anything, I think I'm probably in a better headspace. I'm back in a much more grateful headspace. I've always been a very positive person and I'm not one to let things, you know, get me down. And, I think because of my profile, because of the sort of the attention that the event got, I've realised that I've got to use that now as a platform to try and save more lives. Because if I don't, I don't think I'd be doing other people a service, let alone feeling like I'm being productive – and I like to be productive and helpful to people.*

So, you look at the event that happened and the fact that I was gone for 20 minutes, 25 minutes, with CPR being performed. The chances of surviving were pretty slim. It's only that they did start CPR straight away, and they did very good CPR, and I got through that, and, of course, the AED. But with only, you know, roughly 10 per cent of people surviving, there's not many people who have the profile that I have, who can now use that experience as a platform to help save other lives. So, if I didn't do that, I think I'd feel like I was not really fulfilling my obligations to the community and serving the community in the way that I can. I think I've just got to use it and make something positive happen.

WB Are there any particular things, any specific points or jewels you would like to share?

G *Live every day as if it could be last because you just don't know. At the same time, live it as if you don't want it to be your last. Life is an incredible gift and I absolutely love life. I think life is a creative experience where you get back from it what you put into it. And what you imagine life to be in your head is what it can be. You've just got to make it happen. It doesn't come along and give you it; you've got to create it.*

So, if you want to live an amazing life, you can do it. Live it today because there might not be tomorrow. If there is a tomorrow, make sure it's the best it can be. So, act now and get your heart checked out. Don't have that 1-in-10 chance of surviving a cardiac arrest. That's the only message I would say. Take care of yourself, everybody.

As a result of his cardiac arrest, Greg has a new mission in life, an initiative called Heart of the Nation. He explains:

> *"I believe there is a lack of understanding about AEDs in the community and where you can find them if one is needed. Heart of the Nation is like that Australian Made program with the little logo that goes on Australian-made products."*

Any company, business, community group that has an AED on site can become a member of Heart of the Nation. Stickers are prominently displayed on doors and windows. A Heart of the Nation sticker indicates that location has an AED.

> *"More people need to know about AEDs and know where to find one should a life be endangered. I want to promote that because I've been the beneficiary of an AED working well and I want other people to benefit the same way."*

Heart of the Nation
https://www.heartofthenation.com.au/

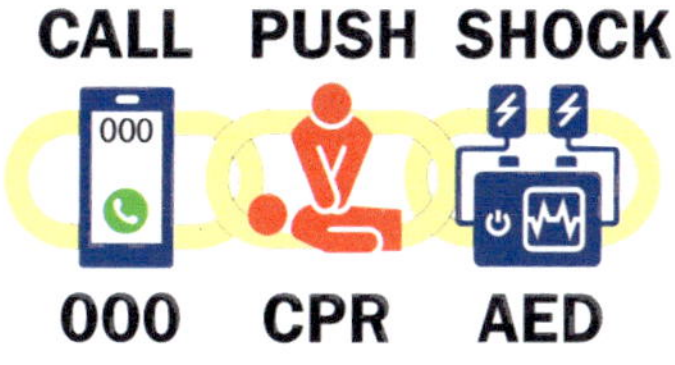

Chain of Survival
https://www.heartofthenation.com.au/chain-of-survival

ANSWERING YOUR QUESTIONS ?

what is a heart attack – an acute myocardial infarction (AMI)?

what is a sudden cardiac arrest (SCA)?

how are they different?

heart attack

As we already know, the term heart attack is a layperson's term and generally refers to an individual having a sudden major heart problem. Most commonly it relates to a sudden blockage of one of the major arteries supplying blood to the heart muscle. Generally, a heart attack leads to pain, sweating, shortness of breath and, sometimes, collapse.

The medical term for a blocked artery that occurs suddenly because of cholesterol plaque is acute myocardial infarction or AMI (*acute* – sudden, *myo* – muscle, *cardial* – of the heart, *infarction* – death caused by lack of blood supply). This medical emergency necessitates the patient being transferred immediately to the nearest hospital to have that artery reopened.

In the event of a heart attack, the person is conscious and breathing.

cardiac arrest

Sometimes, however, the lack of blood flow to the heart muscle can lead to an electrical problem called ventricular fibrillation (*ventricular* – relating to the main pumping chambers of the heart; *fibrillation* – chaotic twitching of muscle fibres). This is a life-threatening sudden cardiac arrest (SCA).

There can be other causes of sudden cardiac arrest that may result in death. These include inherited problems within the heart's electrical system or of the muscle of the heart. This is often experienced as a tragic event, such as a young person collapsing, pulseless, at a sporting event.

A collapsed, pulseless individual needs immediate cardio-pulmonary resuscitation (CPR) – and if available, use of a defibrillator which applies an electric 'shock' to stop the fibrillation and 'restart' the heart. Such action can be lifesaving.

Around the world there are estimated to be more than 1.8 million cardiac arrests per year, including over 800,000 cardiac arrests in Europe and around 33,000 in Australia. Around 60 per cent of patients are unable to be revived by the time the ambulance crew arrives. CPR alone has low rates of effectiveness. However, when provided in combination with defibrillation, survival rates increase significantly.[88]

Early defibrillation is critical for survival from SCA for several reasons[89]:

- the most frequent initial rhythm in witnessed SCA is ventricular fibrillation (VF);
- the treatment for VF is electrical defibrillation;
- the probability of successful defibrillation diminishes rapidly over time;
- VF tends to deteriorate to asystole within a few minutes. Therefore, defibrillation as soon as possible is the standard care for VF.

Defibrillation is effective in over 90 per cent of cases if applied within one minute, but ineffective in over 90 per cent if applied 10 minutes later, even if cardio-pulmonary resuscitation (CPR) is performed[90].

After a cardiac arrest the heart often has electrical activity occurring for about 10 minutes in which, although not beating or pumping blood, the heart 'quivers' with the uncoordinated electrical activity within it. CPR can help get blood to the body, but CPR 'alone' cannot correct this abnormal electrical activity. With each minute that passes after a cardiac arrest, a person loses a 10 per cent survivability chance, meaning there is only a 10-minute window of opportunity to potentially save the person's life.[91]

World-first registry to tackle sudden cardiac death[92] in Australia[93]

19 September 2019

A world-first registry and genetic database is being established in Australia to better understand and prevent sudden cardiac death in young people.

Leading cardiologists, Associate Professor Andre La Gerche from the Baker Heart and Diabetes Institute in Melbourne and Professor Chris Semsarian from the University of Sydney and the Royal Prince Alfred Hospital, are heading this project to aid diagnosis and help establish preventative measures to address the issue of why seemingly fit and healthy people under 50 years die suddenly of cardiac arrest.

The registry will include blood samples from deceased individuals aged up to 50 years affected by sudden cardiac arrest. But perhaps most notably, it will also be the first to include samples of at-risk family members, monitoring clinical assessments, interventions and outcomes in this at-risk population.

State-of-the-art Sudden Cardiac Arrest Clinics have recently opened in Victoria at St Vincent's Hospital and The Alfred Hospital alongside existing clinics at the Royal Melbourne Hospital and Royal Children's Hospital. The clinics will serve as points of contact, support and evaluation for registry participants.

Victoria is the first State to start collecting samples and data, with researchers to work with these leading metropolitan hospitals as well as Ambulance Victoria and the Victorian Institute of Forensic Medicine. Plans are also in place to roll out the initiative in New South Wales, with national implementation to follow.

Head of Sports Cardiology at the Baker Institute, A/Prof. La Gerche says around 25,000 Australians die from sudden cardiac arrest each year, including many young people, and yet we have little insight into how and why this happens.

He says sudden cardiac arrest is the consequence of a number of cardiovascular disorders, with the majority of cases in patients aged less than 50 years and frequently occurring without prior symptoms or warning.

"This highlights the need to discover new mechanisms and markers for early identification of young patients at risk of sudden cardiac arrest," he says.

A/Prof. La Gerche says data from a US registry of sudden death amongst college athletes show cardiovascular causes represent a similar proportion to suicide and drugs combined and exceeded that due to trauma, including car accidents.

Professor Semsarian, a cardiologist who specialises in research looking at genetic heart disease and sudden death, says while there has been no national registry for causes of sudden death up to the age of 50 years in Australia until now, a comparison of multiple databases suggested a similar picture to the US.

"Understanding the precise causes of, and the clinical circumstances and triggers of this, are critical steps in developing targeted clinical and genetic screening programs to prevent sudden cardiac arrest in the community," Prof. Semsarian says.

The primary cause of sudden cardiac death in adults 35 and over is coronary heart disease. In younger people (under 35), it is genetic heart conditions and heart rhythm disorders. Although the rates of heart attacks due to coronary artery disease have decreased significantly over recent decades, the incidence of sudden death in young and middle-aged people has not changed.

IMPORTANT POINTS

- Being fit and living a relatively healthy lifestyle is not necessarily protection against a heart attack.
- Be aware of small signs that could be wrongly attributed to something else, such as 'getting older'.
- There may be no immediate warning of the event itself.
- Cardiac rehabilitation answers the question: "What do I have to do now to keep my heart function well as I move forward?"
- Cardiac rehab has several delivery models. For Greg, it was an at-home, walking program.
- Learn CPR.
- Promote the installation of AEDs within your community or spheres of influence.
- Do not be afraid to use an AED, if necessary, even if you are not trained. The machine tells you what to do. However, you must act quickly.
- Support *Heart of the Nation* if you can do so.

82 *This is an edited version. The full interview can be heard on Dr Bishop's Healthy Heart Network. See page 293 for further details.*

83 *The group, The Wiggles, was founded in 1991 by Anthony Field. Greg Page was a founding member and the original lead singer. He retired in 2006 due to ill health. He made a brief come-back in 2012. Fellow founding members Jeff Fatt and Murray Cook also left in 2012. A new Wiggles lineup, including the fourth original member Anthony Field, debuted at the end of that year. The Wiggles continues today. (The Wiggles: https://www.thewiggles.com)*

84 *ventricular fibrillation is a life-threatening heart arrhythmia in which the bottom chambers of the heart – the ventricles – beat in a rapid and chaotic rhythm*

85 *the ejection fraction (EF) is the amount of blood pumped per beat as a percentage of the total volume of blood in the left ventricle (LV) prior to contraction*

86 *an implantable cardioverter-defibrillator (ICD) detects any life-threatening, rapid heartbeat and shocks the heart back into normal rhythm*

87 *automated external defibrillator (AED) is a sophisticated yet easy-to-use medical device that can analyse the heart's rhythm and, if necessary, deliver an electric shock to help the heart re-establish an effective rhythm*

88 *Lindy Harkness, Lauren Gale, Lara Bishop, Royal Flying Doctor Service (2019), Roll-out of automated external defibrillators to rural and remote Australian communities. 15th National Rural Health Conference, Hobart, Tasmania.*

89 *Ibrahim, Wanis H (2007), Recent advances and controversies in adult cardiopulmonary resuscitation, Postgrad Medical Journal; 83:649–654.*

90 *O'Rourke, M.F (2010) Reality of Out of Hospital Cardiac Arrest, BMJ Journals.*

91 *op. cit. Lindy Harkness, Lauren Gale, Lara Bishop*

92 *Sudden cardiac death — also sudden cardiac arrest and unexplained cardiac death — is one of the biggest killers of Australians under 50 and is five times more likely to affect men. The primary cause of SCD in adults 35 and over is coronary heart disease. In younger people (under 35) it is congenital heart conditions and heart rhythm disorders. Many of the younger people affected by SCD are generally regarded as being fit and healthy and we have little information on why the problem occurs. In Australia the rates of SCD in people aged under 35 years are thought to be 1 in 30,000 (Semsarian et al. New England Journal of Medicine 2016), and in middle-aged people is it likely to be a least twice this figure. [https://baker.edu.au/health hub/sudden-cardiac-death]*

93 *Baker Heart and Diabetes Institute media release: https://baker.edu.au/news/mediareleases/ sudden-cardiac-death-registry*

Too many cardiac event sufferers become 'repeat offenders'. Maintenance, monitoring and a healthy heart lifestyle help keep everyone living a healthier life.

chapter 17

MAINTENANCE AND PREVENTION

You met Ron in the introduction to this book. In 2018, aged 66, he was living what seemed a healthy life. Yet, annual blood tests showed that his total cholesterol persistently hovered over 6. His GP reassured him that, despite this, given the combination of the other circumstances of his life, he needn't worry.

Ron continues ...

PATIENT'S PERSPECTIVE

an unwelcome interruption disrupts an ordered life

On a Monday morning in August 2018, I had a heart attack. I was eating breakfast when a dull ache commenced in my chest and became progressively a more painful crushing sensation. The pain was a strong pressure pain, not sharp or stabbing and, at first, not too agonising.

It took a few minutes for me to start worrying that this was more than a serious bout of indigestion and possibly a heart attack.

As an unfortunate result of the influence of news reports in the previous few days that ambulance ramping at the Royal Hobart Hospital meant that ambulances were delayed in responding to calls, I phoned for a taxi. During the taxi ride to the hospital, I had the sensation of both my arms from the shoulders down feeling progressively cold and deadened in sensation. I wondered, somewhat disassociated from what was happening, if this was the feeling of my body dying.

When I arrived at the Emergency Department, the swift response to my symptoms belied the frequent news reports of long waits in ED. I was placed on a gurney, surrounded by medical staff, given some medication to swallow and fitted with various apparatus. While constantly being asked to rate my chest pain from 1 to 10, I was wheeled to another floor where I was taken in for an angiogram. A catheter device was threaded into my wrist and up into the arteries around my heart. Projected onto a TV screen I was able to see the resulting grey spidery images of blockages and near blockages in several arteries, as the cardiologist explained what they were. One artery was quite blocked, and three others were nearly blocked. ...

I underwent various tests ... The team of cardiologists and surgeons considered the alternative treatments of the use of stents or coronary artery bypass surgery (CABG). Because of the number of arteries that were blocked or imminently blocked, surgery was chosen. ...

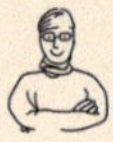

While this is Ron's retelling of his experience, calling triple zero is the recommended action.

Ron's surgery was successful, and he underwent the cardiac rehabilitation program he describes in the Introduction.

three years later ...

Once the hospital organised rehabilitation program was completed, there was no further hospital supported rehabilitation. However, my rehabilitation after heart surgery didn't come to an end after the conclusion of the hospital program. My energy and strength took about another six months to return to something resembling my pre-heart attack state.

The cardiac rehabilitation nurses had warned that many times they witnessed the return of patients as early as a year after their last hospitalisation for heart surgery. In many cases this was the result of patients failing to take on board the heart health information and advice they had received. I realised that it was not just a matter of rehabilitation, presumably back to a reasonable state of health, but of maintaining that state of health.

In my case, even considering what I had learned during the cardiac rehabilitation program, there was little that I could identify that I needed to change in my lifestyle. Prior to my heart attack, the only indication that something could be wrong was that my cholesterol reading, which had always hovered in the mid-4s for years, had increased to the mid-6s in the previous few years. Because none of the other warning signs such as being overweight, smoking, diabetes applied to me, my GP had assured me that there was nothing to be concerned about. Nevertheless, at that time I decreased my consumption of red meat to almost nil, decreased my dairy intake and reduced it to low fat products and continued regular hour long walks most days of the week. So, even after having a heart attack, there seemed little more I could do, beside take the medications I was now prescribed. I became just a little more rigorous in observing my diet and further reduced my alcohol consumption to a glass or two of wine every few weeks rather than every weekend.

Having completed cardiac rehabilitation with no clear answers as to how I had ended up with heart disease, I was troubled by the 'injustice' of it all. I tried to account for how it came about. I wondered if stress had somehow been the contributing factor. About the time that my cholesterol reading increased, I had to negotiate placing my mother in a nursing home, and in a distant city from where I live. At about the same time, my son was diagnosed with a slow moving but terminal brain tumour requiring surgery and my daughter cut off all contact with me. These circumstances prevailed for a couple of years and then my mother died. At the same time, my son's brain tumour reappeared, no longer operable but requiring radiation and chemotherapy treatment. Could these circumstances have contributed to my heart disease? There was no way of knowing, but I gave more attention to meditation and taking things calmly. One positive outcome of my heart attack was that it brought my daughter (and grandchildren) back into my life. And surprisingly, being overtly confronted with my mortality has made me more accepting of life's circumstances.

And so, today, I continue living as healthily as I can. Nevertheless, I live with a heightened sense of my mortality, that awareness more pronounced when I experience the occasional twinges of pain or discomfort in my chest. At such times, I wonder, Is my heart about to suffer another attack? Will this be the end game? *To be prepared, I have done the necessary organisational things such as updating my will, setting up power of attorney, organising finances so as not to leave behind too much of a mess for others to clean up. Otherwise, I just try to get on with life.*

- Ron, Hobart, Tasmania, Australia

prevention

Keeping your heart healthy is something to be worked on every day.

The key elements to a healthy lifestyle are:

- what you eat and drink
  - this is not a diet but your pattern of eating over days, weeks and months ...
- how much you move
  - daily movement is essential; be aware of how much sitting you do in a day
- how well you sleep
- if you are a smoker or not
  - quitting smoking has an almost immediate positive effect on your risk of heart attack or stroke
  - be aware of the dangers of passive smoking
- how you control your cholesterol and blood pressure
  - if the doctor recommends medication, take it as prescribed, for as long as prescribed
  - know your numbers and have them checked regularly
  - have a good relationship with your cardiologist / doctor / pharmacist / other health care providers
  - ask questions; engage with your health carers
- understand the impact of stress and be mindful of what you can do to minimise it
- ensure that you have good support for a balanced lifestyle from your family and friends.

family

Cardiac rehabilitation offers an opportunity to extend the investigation to the wider family. As part of the recovery from a heart related event, the cardiologist has an opportunity to pose the question, *If this has happened to you, could it happen to someone else in your family?* One way to answer the question is through cardiac imaging, a precise investigation into the health of a person's heart, regardless of risk factors and population data percentages.

Dr Warrick:

A female patient of mine had agreed that her partner, who had heart disease in the family, should be checked. However, he died from a heart attack before he came to see me. This is a reminder of how dangerous coronary artery disease can be and how almost anyone could be at risk.

IMPORTANT POINTS

- A healthy life into the future is not just about recovering from the heart event. It requires detailed attention to maintaining a good state of health – after **and** before an event or diagnosis.
- Now could be the time to consider having your family members see a GP for a heart check
  - and if indicated, a heart scan.

chapter 18

REHAB FOR LIFE

YOUR DIY REHAB PROGRAM – FOR LIFE

your rehab journey - important information

take this information to appointments with your doctors

(ask your cardiac doctors or nurses for help to fill in this section)

type of heart event *(please circle)*

heart attack   cardiac arrest   cardiac failure

valve problem

aortic   mitral   tricuspid   pulmonary

reason/s if known

date of event(s)

procedure or intervention *(please circle)*

stenting:	number of stents	1	2	more
	artery(ies) impacted	LAD	Circumflex	RCA

cardiothoracic surgery:

	bypass grafting	number of grafts ____________		
		LIMA	RIMA	SVG
	valve surgery	aortic	mitral	tricuspid
		pulmonary	metallic or tissue	

---

other medical history

high blood pressure			
family history (men less than 55 / women less than 60)			
smoking	past	current	
over ideal weight	little	moderately	significantly
diabetes or raised blood sugar			
renal impairment	mild	moderate	severe
atrial fibrillation	type		
cardiac failure	type		
other major conditions *(please specify)*			

MEDICATION LIST

drug	dose	frequency	action of the drug

MEDICATION LIST

drug	dose	frequency	action of the drug

MEDICATION LIST

drug	dose	frequency	action of the drug

top tips for taking your medicines

Always follow your doctor's or pharmacist's advice on taking your heart medicines. If you are not happy about any aspect of your medication regime, please talk with your doctor or pharmacist, and, if you are still not happy, seek a second option. **Do not self-medicate or self-diagnose.** Remember[94]:

- **Keep taking your medicines** even if you feel well. Only stop or change the dose of your medicines on the advice of your doctor.
- Talk to your doctor or pharmacist about **possible side-effects**. Understand what you should do if you suffer side-effects.
- Check with your doctor or pharmacist before taking any **over-the-counter medicines**. Over-the-counter medicines are medicines you can buy from a pharmacy, supermarket or health food shop without a prescription. These include pain medicines, cold and flu medicines, supplements and vitamins. They can interact with heart medicines or can make your heart condition worse.
- Check with your doctor or pharmacist if there are **any foods or drinks you should avoid** as some can interact with heart medicines.
- Ensure you **always have enough supply** of your medicines.
- **Keep a list of your medicines with you at all times**; either written down *(see previous page)* or on your phone. Take this list to all your health appointments.
- **Check the expiry date.** Only take medicines that are within their expiry date.
- **Only take medicines that have been prescribed for you**. Never share your medicines with anyone nor take someone else's.

For a free downloadable printable PDF version of these REHAB FOR LIFE pages, please visit the Healthy Heart Network: https://drwarrickbishop.com/page/cardiac-rehab-bookbonuses

YOUR REHAB JOURNEY - THE 3 Es

education

exercise

emotional support

*Most rehab programs run for between six and 10 weeks. However, we believe **the journey is for life** and want you to embrace your second chance at life – for life.*

education

We suggest you re-read material from this book frequently.

- Remind yourself of what may have led to your situation in the first place.
- What can you do to avoid a future event?
- Do you know what medications you are on? (*Ensure the table on page 249 is filled out correctly.)*
- Do you understand why you are on your medications?
- Do you have new medications?
    - Have you added these to your list?
    - Have you deleted any that you are no longer taking?
- Do you have medications that can be stopped?
    - dual antiplatelet therapy (DAPT), for example.

We also suggest ongoing education[95]:

- www.healthyheartnetwork.com
    - our Know Your Real Risk of Heart Attack Facebook group
    - our podcasts
    - our blogs
    - membership of the Healthy Heart Network

- Healthy Heart Network courses
  - weight loss
  - atrial fibrillation
  - cardiac failure
- our books
  - *Atrial Fibrillation Explained*
  - *Cardiac Failure Explained*
  - *Have You Planned Your Heart Attack?*
  - *Know Your Real Risk of Heart Attack*
  - more books to come.

exercise

on discharge from hospital / after diagnosis

We highly recommend that you attend a rehab program endorsed by the hospital where you have been a patient, or your cardiologist.

If this is not possible due to circumstances such as living in an isolated area, we suggest the following, undertaken in consultation with your medical team.

each session

start with a 5-to-10-minute warm up

- gentle walking, gentle stationary bike cycling, gentle marching on the spot
- gentle stretching

exercise session

PLEASE - REMEMBER TO GO SLOWLY!

we suggest walking

- using 'easy talking' as the guide to activity intensity
  - if you are puffed as you walk and talk, you are going too fast
  - if you are not puffed at all, you can increase the intensity a little and test yourself
- time yourself and aim to reach 40 minutes
- try to measure distance
  - laps of an oval, park or similar venue
  - many watches and fitness apps measure distance in steps, kilometres, and/or miles

we **do not**

- focus on heart rate, as the medications can often confuse this
- use effort score as this tends to become a competition

end with a 5-to-10-minute cool down

- gentle walking, gentle stationary bike cycling, gentle marching on the spot
- gentle stretching

after your organised rehab program / your self-directed gentle program at home

exercise regularly for the remainder of your life

- current recommendations are 30+ mins x 5 or more times per week – incorporating both aerobic and strengthening activities
- find something you enjoy doing so that you will turn it into a habit
- walking is always an excellent option

recording your effort is important (you manage what you measure)

- fill in the days you are able to exercise
- total your week's exercise distance to see your progress

REMEMBER: take this information to appointments with your doctor

	last week's time/steps/distance	Monday	Tuesday	Wed.	Thurs.	Friday	Sat.	Sunday
wk 1	0							
wk 2								
wk 3								
wk 4								
wk 5								
wk 6								

emotional support

We suggest you

- speak with your spouse/partner and other significant people in your life about your changed health circumstances and ask them to speak with you regularly about how you are coping and feeling
- raise any emotional issues at your doctor's appointments
- list the people you will need to help you on your journey, recognising that some of these people will change along the way:

spouse / partner

significant other / carer

general practitioner

surgeon

cardiologist

rehab nurse

dietician

physical trainer

other professionals

other family members

friends

Join here: https://healthyheartnetwork.come/page/fb-group

94 *based on material from the (Australian) Heart Foundation website: https://www.heartfoundation.org.au/Recovery-and-support/Taking-your-medicine*

95 *please see page 294 for access to these powerfully supportive resources*

epilogue

A MIRACULOUS JOURNEY

Not in my wildest dreams did I consider that when Alistair and I started to formulate the basis for this book, at the time of reading the final draft, I would be a beneficiary of its contents.

Amazingly, ironically, surprisingly, and out of the blue, 18 months ago I discovered that my heart had a problem – a dilated ascending aorta.

Five weeks ago to the day as I write this, I had open-heart surgery to correct the problem. Wow!

My journey of discovery and my experience through surgery will contribute to a newly planned book, likely to be called *Open Heart Surgery Explained.* Importantly, though, it is the rehab journey that I want to touch on here. Well-researched and highly encouraged knowledge has become my firsthand experience.

My rehabilitation journey began as soon as the surgical date was set.

Although I have always been a fit person, I upped the intensity of my exercise to be as fit as possible. I saw my GP to ensure my bloods were okay. I ate well and even started meditation. I wanted to have as many things in my favour as possible when I went under the knife.

After the surgery I experienced fear – pain – uncertainty – discomfort irregular bowels – an acute sense of frailty. For years I have sent numerous people for open-heart surgery. Now I **know**!

The first few days following the surgery are a bit of a blur, and I have to say I was, perhaps, not as brave as others, wallowing a little in self-pity. A defining moment came on day two when my surgeon **strongly** encouraged me to get out of bed in an effort to 'normalise' to a pre-morbid existence. With his stern encouragement ringing in my ears, I made every effort to be out of bed and moving as much as possible. I certainly didn't want him to catch me in bed again!

Six days after surgery I walked out of The Prince Charles Hospital (Brisbane, Queensland) and haven't stopped walking. Since my return to Hobart, I've been seen by my local doctor, in touch with my cardiologist and have had follow-up with the local cardiac rehab team who are providing support and guidance towards my recovery.

I'm about two weeks away from returning to work. I will ease into this gradually and check in with my GP regularly.

I'm not back to 'normal' yet. I still have discomfort in my chest and a desperate fear of sneezing because of the pain. Having said that, five weeks into the post-operative journey, when I now look forward, I can clearly see the path to returning to a new 'normal'.

If you have experienced open-heart surgery, I can genuinely empathise with you. I truly wish your journey will be as smooth and quick as possible.

While we all travel different paths, there are some constants: our loved ones who travel beside us, the amazing medical team who gets us through the surgery, our GP, and, of course, our rehabilitation team. And a miraculous journey unfolds.

Wishing that you live as well as possible for as long as possible.

Warrick Bishop,
Hobart, Tasmania, Australia
11 October 2022

APPENDICES

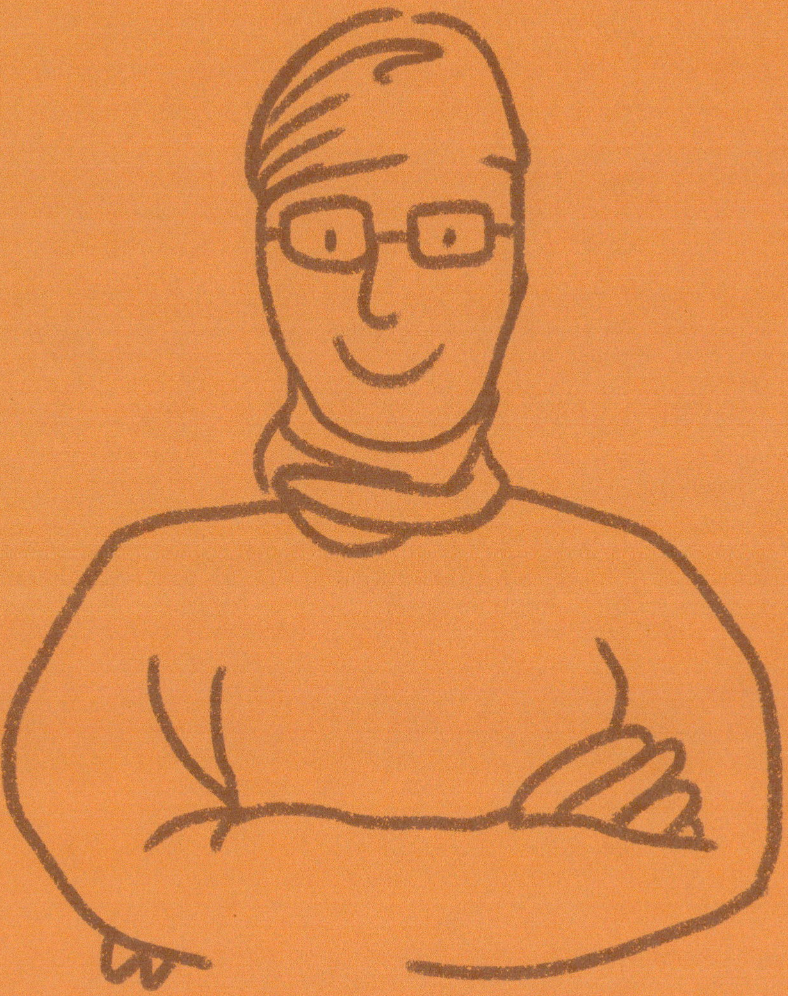

appendix 1

WILL YOU RECOGNISE A HEART ATTACK?[96]

Will you recognise your heart attack?

Heart Foundation

Warning Signs Action Plan

Do you feel any

pain | pressure | heaviness | tightness

In one or more of your

chest | neck | jaw | arm/s | back | shoulder/s

You may also feel

nauseous | a cold sweat | dizzy | short of breath

Yes

1 STOP and rest now

2 TALK tell someone how you feel

If you take angina medicine

- Take a dose of your medicine.
- Wait 5 minutes. Still have symptoms? Take another dose of your medicine.
- Wait 5 minutes. Symptoms won't go away?

Are your symptoms severe or getting worse?

or

Have your symptoms lasted 10 minutes?

Yes

3 CALL 000 Triple Zero

and chew 300mg aspirin, unless you have an allergy to aspirin or your doctor has told you not to take it

- Ask for an ambulance.
- Don't hang up.
- Wait for the operator's instructions.

appendix 2
MORE ABOUT VALVES

In the main text of this book, we wrote about the importance of the one-way valves that keep the blood flowing in the right direction through the heart.

The first of these, the **tricuspid** valve allows the oxygen-poor, dark purple, carbon dioxide-rich blood to move from the right atrium into the right ventricle. The ventricle then pumps the blood through another one-way valve, the **pulmonary** valve, into the lungs where the blood becomes replenished with fresh oxygen. Bright red, oxygen-rich blood then flows from the lungs through the four pulmonary veins into the left atrium which pumps the blood through the **mitral** valve into the left ventricle. The left ventricle then contracts, squeezing blood through the **aortic** valve into the main artery of the body, the aorta.

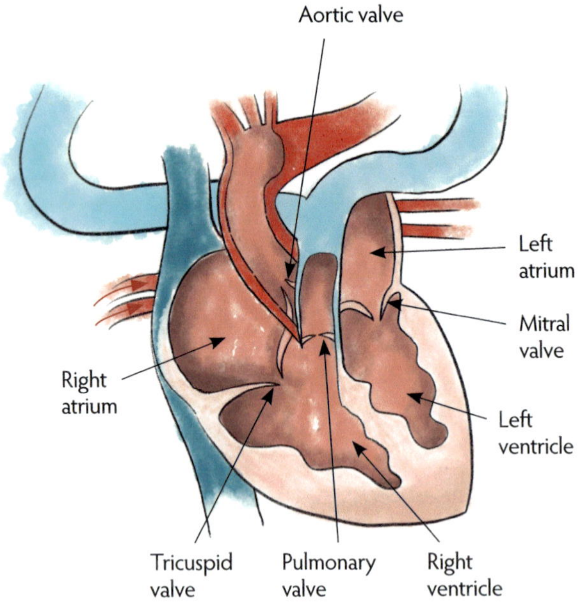

valves of the heart

These valves act like tightly closed doors that stop the blood flowing in the wrong direction. Healthy valves are important for good heart function, maximising pump efficiency so the heart can function throughout a life-time. The human heart pumps around 100,000 times a day. Each time the heart beats valves open and close to allow the blood to flow.

100,000 times a day x 7 days a week x 52 weeks a year x 80, 90 or even 100 years = well over 3 billion heart beats! How fantastic is that?

valvular heart disease

Valves, like everything else, can have problems, too.

They can be tight and affect ‘forward’ flow, or they can leak and allow the blood to flow ‘backwards’ in the wrong direction. Should any one of the heart’s valves – the aortic, the mitral, the pulmonary or the tricuspid valve – have a problem, such as being tight and limiting forward flow, or leaking and allowing reverse flow, it has an impact on the circulation. In the forward direction, it affects **pressure** while in the reverse direction, it causes **congestion**.

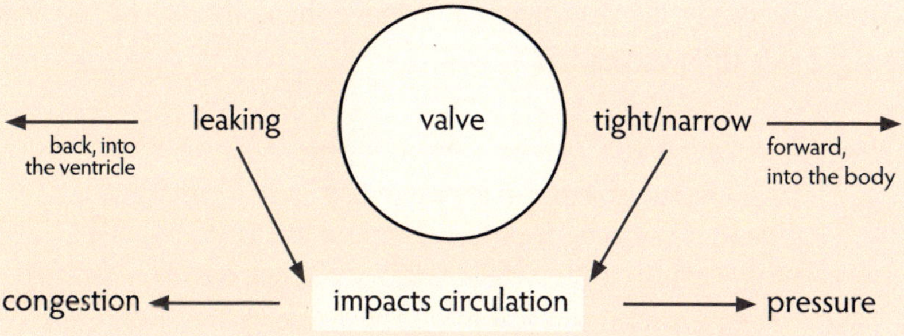

Imagine that the aortic valve is too narrow. The left ventricle needs to pump harder to get the blood out of the heart and into the body. The result is similar to the person having high blood pressure.

What if the valve leaks, so that every time the ventricle pumps blood out, some leaks back in, lessening the amount of blood pumped around the body? The heart tries to accommodate by dilating the left ventricle, increasing its size so that it pumps a higher volume of blood into the circulation. While some of the blood regurgitates into the left ventricle, enough is pumped into the circulatory system to meet the body’s requirements.

most common

The most common cause of valvular heart disease in western communities is associated with ageing and presents as a degenerative disease of the left-sided aortic and mitral valves.

The **aortic valve**, the outlet valve of the heart, is the one most replaced. It has three cusps, and these cusps can become stiff and fused with age, causing **aortic stenosis**. Some people are born with only two cusps in the valve and they may require a valve replacement at an earlier age, around 60 years old.

Less commonly, the aortic valve is replaced due to a leakage, known as **regurgitation**, often associated with high blood pressure. Regurgitation is often behind replacement of the **mitral valve,** the other major valve affected in valvular heart disease.

The right-sided heart valves, the pulmonary and tricuspid valves, are rarely replaced because the right side of the heart has fairly low-pressure circulation. Generally, also the heart can cope more easily with a leaky valve on the right side than on the left.

Valvular heart disease is generally not hereditary. However, some cases of aortic stenosis can be hereditary – when a valve has only two cusps and it wears out prematurely. Should anyone in your family have valvular heart disease, it would be wise to have a discussion with your general practitioner or a consultation with a cardiologist.

symptoms

The earliest and most common symptom of the valvular heart disease is shortness of breath on exertion. If the aortic valve is narrowed, and is in a more advanced stage of impairment, it can also give rise to episodes of dizziness and chest pain on exertion. The mitral valve, likewise, tends to give rise to shortness of breath when the leak becomes more advanced.

Narrowing of the mitral valve can also lead to shortness of breath. Mitral valve disease also commonly produces palpitations, and less commonly gives rise to chest discomfort or dizziness. Some mild degree of dysfunction of the valve can be tolerated, but more severe valve disease causes the symptoms.

diagnosis

While valvular heart disease can be diagnosed by discussing a patient's history together with a clinical examination, **an echocardiogram** (echo) **is the diagnostic test** of choice to determine the presence or absence of any valvular heart disease. The working capacity of each valve can be assessed individually. Determining flow through the valves helps ascertain pressures within the heart and the valves themselves. Velocity assessment is used to calculate pressures within the heart and this, too, becomes vital data. The echo is also useful for following up patients to assess the progress of the disease to determine if the valve(s) needs to be repaired or replaced.

WHAT IS A HEART MURMUR?

A heart murmur is the sound of blood passing through the heart across the heart valves. It may be benign in which case the heart is normal and the murmur is merely due to audible flow, or 'turbulence', across the heart valves. Some murmurs can come and go because of certain conditions associated with an increase in the heart pumping capacity, for example pregnancy, infection, thyroid over activity, anaemia. Some murmurs are due to a problem with the heart itself, such as a leaky or narrow valve. Less commonly, a murmur may be due to a hole in the heart.

Australian cardiology first gives Nadeane new lease on life[98]

Interventional cardiologist duo Dr Karl Poon and Dr Dale Murdoch had just 10 seconds to save the life of patient Nadeane Giles in a complex Australian-first heart procedure at The Prince Charles Hospital.

Suffering from mitral stenosis – a severe narrowing of her mitral heart valve – 73-year-old Nadeane's health was ailing as she was left breathless and unable to walk to her letterbox. All efforts to treat her condition had been rendered unsuitable, with medication exhausted and three surgeons advising open-heart surgery was not possible – leaving Nadeane only one option, to take a gamble on a never-before-attempted mitral valve procedure.

Nadeane's treating team comprising Dr Karl Poon and Dr Dale Murdoch rose to the challenge, spending several months undertaking extensive 3D planning and consulting with colleagues around the globe before tackling the complex procedure in March 2020.

Dr Poon said he had explained to Nadeane the process would be high risk, as her heart would be temporarily stopped while the team remotely placed a new heart valve in the mitral position.

"We were granted just 10 seconds to remotely place the valve in the mitral space within millimetre accuracy while her heart was stopped. However, if the valve was incorrectly placed or sized, this would be the difference between life and death," Dr Poon said.

"This high-risk procedure involves inserting a heart valve through the groin into the middle of the heart without any open chest surgery – the first time in Australia this has been done for the mitral valve position."

Eight cardiologists and three hours later, Nadeane was out of theatre and immediately experiencing an improvement in her health.

"I knew this procedure was my only chance to live and I was going to take it and run with it," Ms Giles said.

And run with it she has, returning home to enjoy riding her bike, walking and planning plenty of travel around Australia.

Dr Murdoch said there was an overwhelming sense of relief and excitement when the valve was successfully placed with the aid of expert cardiac imaging performed by TPCH's Clinical Director Echocardiography Professor Greg Scalia.

Their collective efforts showed results within 30 seconds.

"There was more than 20 of us in the room, and we were so happy to achieve this result for Nadeane, as we could see the heart waking up in front of our eyes," Dr Murdoch said.

"The success of this procedure now opens doors for dozens of other patients just like Nadeane, who have been unable to be helped so far."

Dr Poon and Dr Murdoch have been praised internationally by colleagues and peers for their skill and commitment to successfully completing the procedure, but nobody has higher praise for the team than Nadeane.

"I'll be forever grateful for my second chance," Ms Giles said.

appendix 3

MORE ABOUT ATRIAL FIBRILLATION

Atrial fibrillation occurs when electrical impulses in the upper chambers of the heart, the atria, become chaotic, and instead of producing a steady, regular beat, they generate a scattered irregular, very fast and uncontrolled heartbeat. These impulses from the chaotic atria transmit to the ventricles, and their beat, too, becomes irregularly irregular. As a result, the heart does not pump properly.

AF is common after cardiac surgery.

People often present with the classic symptom of palpitation which can be accompanied by a range of symptoms including lack of energy, breathlessness, dizziness, chest tightness, poor appetite, swelling of the ankles. When the heart doesn't pump well, blood can stagnate inside the atria and clot. If the clot breaks away and travels to the brain, it causes a stroke.

Unfortunately, while it is an increasingly common condition, many people are unaware of having it as AF can be asymptomatic – and it is found as an incidental finding (when, the patient is undergoing a health check, or is being treated for another condition) or when the person presents with a devastating stroke.

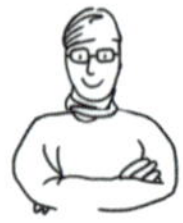

The two common causes of stroke are AF and high blood pressure. Thinning the blood using appropriate medication is well accepted as a means of reducing an AF sufferer's risk of stroke back toward that of the general community. Detection and proper treatment of AF are extremely important, as is the monitoring of blood pressure.

When a person presents with similar symptoms as outlined above, the cardiologist will look at the cardiac risk factors, which, as we have already seen with coronary artery disease, include genetics and family history, and numerous lifestyle factors.

While the genetic factors associated with AF are not well understood, some genes are known to cause AF. Family history, particularly where sufferers have been younger and especially when coupled with no other obvious AF triggers, is also another strong indicator.

the big '3'

Age is an unavoidable AF risk factor, as are cardiac surgery and other major surgeries.

However, **high blood pressure**, **obesity** and **alcohol** are the 'big 3' of a number of modifiable risk factors.

High blood pressure causes pressure changes within the heart that can stretch the left atrium. Over time, this stretching changes the shape of the atrium, increasing the likelihood of it developing an abnormal rhythm, and in particular, AF.

Obesity is firmly established as an independent risk factor in the incidence and progression of AF. Associated with obesity is **poor sleep** and especially sleep apnoea, in which a person's sleep is interrupted when the airway closes due to too much weight around the throat. When a person doesn't have an obvious cause for AF, sleep apnoea is a good place to start the exploration.

Alcohol is the third significant lifestyle risk factor. Studies involving teetotallers and drinkers have shown a direct link between the amount of alcohol consumed and the risk for atrial fibrillation. For anyone who is susceptible to AF, every drink consumed increases the risk.

how AF shows up – if at all

Atrial fibrillation manifests in one of two ways:

- **overt** (symptomatic) AF
  - in which the patient feels palpitations in the chest, an irregularity, a fluttering, which is described quite clearly. Shortness of breath on exertion, for example while climbing the stairs or carrying the groceries, and a decrease in exercise capacity may also be experienced. Because AF can occur very suddenly, and because the heart is not pumping normally, it can also be associated with low blood pressure and patients may present with a collapse,
- **silent** (asymptomatic) AF
  - the type of which the patient is not aware, and it is discovered as an accidental finding, for example, during a regular blood pressure check.

AF is also referred to in terms of time the patient is in the abnormal rhythm:

- **paroxysmal** (between 24 - 48 hours but no longer than a week)
- **persistent** (present longer than seven days)
- **permanent** (present for longer than a year).

diagnosis

Diagnosis is confirmed through the results of an **electrocardiogram** (ECG) which measures the electrical activity of the heart. In a healthy heart, the ECG shows sinus rhythm, a beautiful synchronous atrial contraction

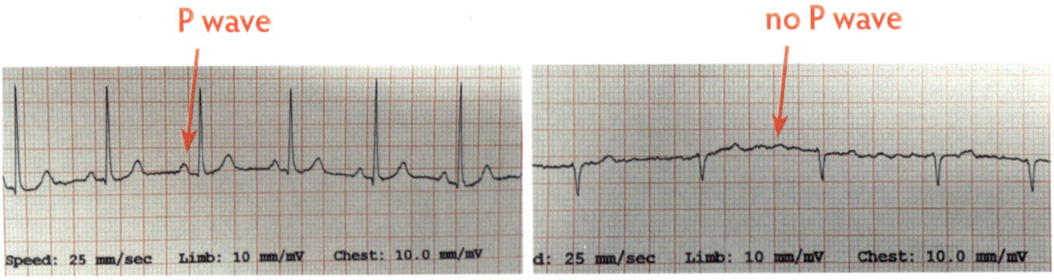

ECG diagnosis of atrial fibrillation: left, sinus rhythm; right, atrial fibrillation

followed by a beautiful synchronous ventricle contraction. In AF, the atria lose their synchronicity; the beats become chaotic and irregular. In a normal ECG, a P-wave is followed by a QRS and a T wave. In AF, **there is no P-wave;** this is its diagnostic thumb print.

management

Once diagnosed, AF needs management to reduce the risk of recurrence and of the condition itself, in terms of symptoms and prognosis.

The number one risk is the person having a stroke. Blood pooling in a left atrium that is not contracting properly can lead to the formation of a clot in the left atrial appendage. Should this clot dislodge, it can pass through the left ventricle, make its way to the brain, and cause a stroke. Stroke is a devastating consequence of AF.

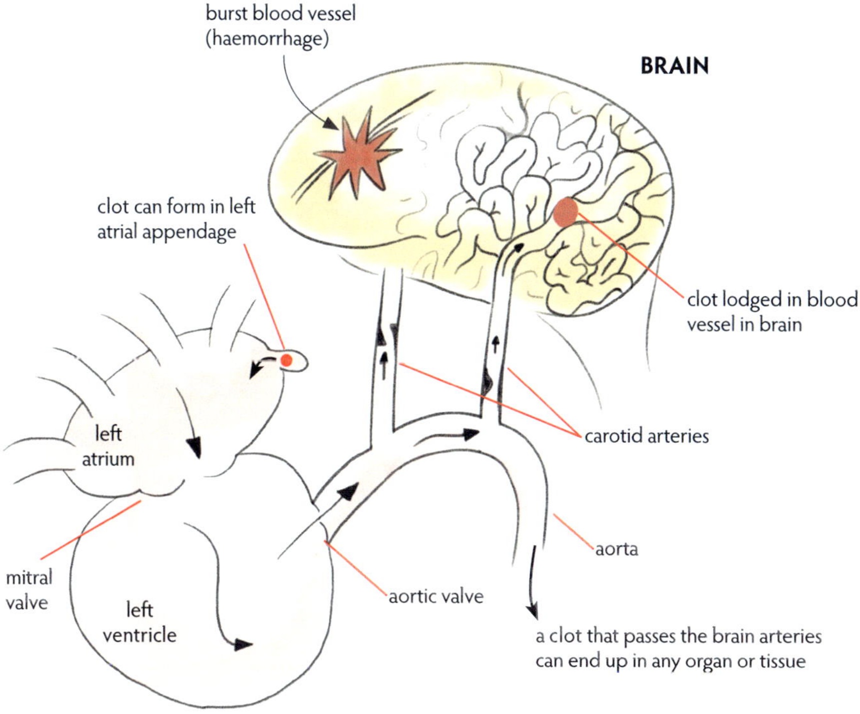

origins of a stroke

However, the risk of a stroke needs to be weighed against the risk of bleeding as a consequence of the patient taking blood thinners. A risk score calculator has been developed for each consideration, the CHA2DS2-VA score (risk of having a stroke) and the HAS-BLED score (risk of bleeding). *(see the next page for further details)*

When it comes to treatment, an assessment is made about whether or not a patient should take a blood thinner to reduce the risk of stroke – even if there are no symptoms. Decisions are also made around correcting the heart rhythm, controlling the heart rate, and treating complications, such as a build-up of fluid which could worsen shortness of breath. Lifestyle advice is given about weight, alcohol, and exercise.

WHAT IS A NORMAL HEART RHYTHM?

The heart's normal, healthy rhythm is called ***sinus rhythm*** *because it is controlled by the sinoatrial, or sinus, node. In a healthy heart, this beating occurs in a synchronistic and smooth manner. Visualise, if you can, a squid moving through the water. Synchronous. Coordinated. Smooth. When this synchronicity breaks down, arrhythmia occurs. One of the most common forms of heart arrhythmia is atrial fibrillation which, according to the European Society of Cardiology (ESC), is one of the major causes of stroke, heart failure, sudden death, and cardiovascular disease in the world. The ESC also predicts that its prevalence will rise steeply in coming years.*

A CLOSER LOOK

keeping score

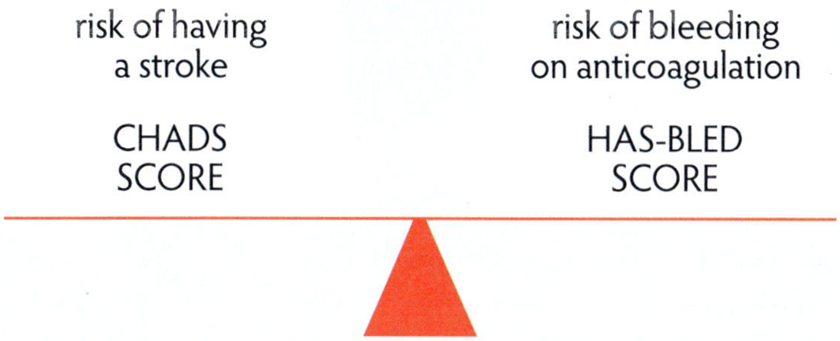

balancing risks

People who suffer **C**ardiac failure, high blood pressure (**H**ypertension), increasing **A**ge, **D**iabetes and previous **S**troke (CHADS) have an increased risk of stroke if they also have atrial fibrillation. A tool has been formulated in which these parameters receive a score, the tally of which is then used in management decisions. The original CHADS score has been modified with more information being added.

Today's CHA2DS2-VA score offers extra options: age variability (it breaks down age groups into lower, intermediate and higher risks), the patient's sex (women run a higher risk of stroke), and it also adds, as a consideration, previous stroke or vascular disease within the arterial system. As these parameters provide a likelihood of the risk of stroke in the future, the score is used in decision-making regarding the need for anticoagulation therapy.

The question is then asked, *How safe is anticoagulant therapy for that patient?* with the consideration here being the risk of bleeding.

Another score has been developed, HAS-BLED: **H**ypertension, **A**bnormal renal or liver function, previous **S**troke, previous **B**leeding problems principally from the gut, **L**abile control of warfarin (labile INR), **E**lderly (over 65 years of age), **D**rugs or alcohol. Again, each parameter is given a score, with the tally indicating the risk of bleeding for that individual.

The CHA2DS2-VA score and the HAS-BLED score are married to help

The HAS-BLED score was developed before the Non-vitamin K Oral AntiCoagulant [NOAC] agents became widely available and so the labile INR can be removed from the score if a NOAC is to be used. However, if that is done, the medical practitioner needs to consider renal function as this is known to be a driver for risk of bleeding. Adequate renal function is needed for metabolism of the NOACs and if renal function reduces, the NOAC dosage needs to be adjusted down.

to make a management decision for the patient, weighing up the risks for the person the best way possible. The risks need to be reviewed periodically as both scores can change with time. For example, the age component will increase, the cardiac failure component could change, high blood pressure could be brought under control or develop.

Although these scores are dynamic, they give a good understanding for trying to mitigate future risk of stroke and future risk of bleeding for the patient.

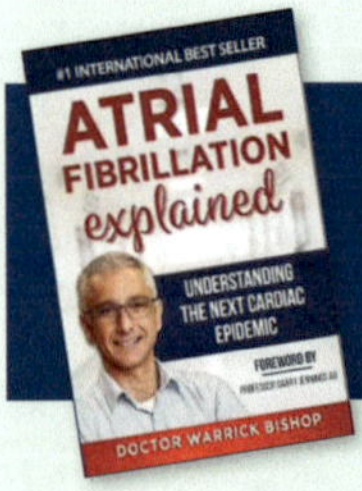

For further information on atrial fibrillation, please refer to Dr Bishop's book, *Atrial Fibrillation Explained* (see page 295 for details)

appendix 4

RECIPES[103]

BREAKFAST

acai smoothie bowl

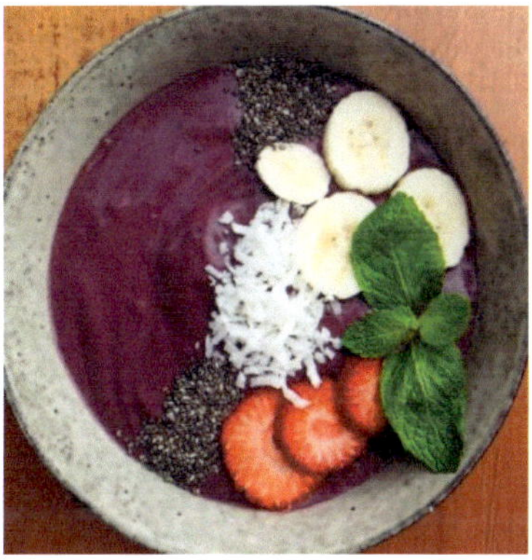

SERVINGS: 1

PREP TIME: 2 mins

serving suggestion

Serve with chopped strawberries, fresh mint, shredded coconut, chia seeds.

ingredients

100 g frozen Acai puree

½ frozen banana

¼ cup coconut milk

method

Blitz all ingredients in a blender until smooth but remaining thick.

Pour into a serving bowl and decorate.

granola

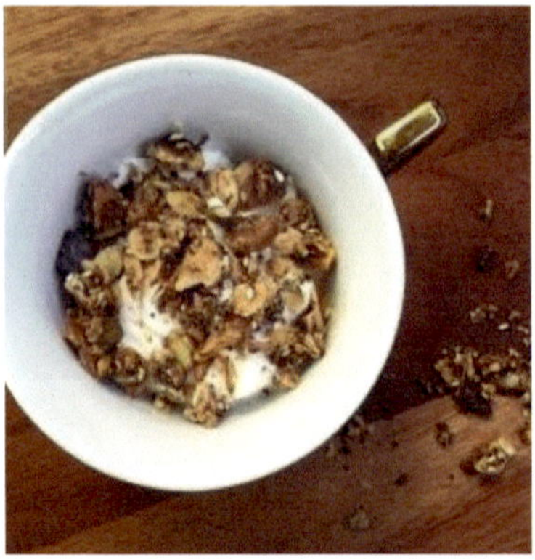

SERVINGS: 8

PREP TIME: 10 mins

COOKING TIME: 40 mins

serving suggestion

Serve the granola with berries, cream and/or full fat, unsweetened Greek or natural yoghurt.

ingredients

2 tsp coconut oil

2 tsp ground cinnamon

2 tbsp ground ginger

75 g walnuts, roughly chopped

50 g macadamias

50 g flaked almonds

50 g pumpkin seeds/pepitas

50 g sunflower seeds

25 g flax/linseeds

1 tsp vanilla bean extract

100 g shaved coconut

method

Preheat the oven to 160°C and line two baking trays with baking paper.

Melt the coconut oil over a medium heat, then add the cinnamon and ginger and stir to release the fragrances.

Add the nuts and seeds and stir until well coated, then remove the pan from the heat and stir through the vanilla bean extract.

Spread the mixture evenly across the trays, then bake for 10-15 minutes, stirring every 5 minutes to prevent the mixture from burning.

Remove the trays from the oven, then reduce the heat to 120°C.

Add the shaved coconut and stir to combine, then return the trays to the oven for another 10-15 minutes, or until the granola is dried through. Alternatively, turn the oven off after 10 minutes and leave the granola in the oven to dry for another 30-40 minutes.

storage

Store in an airtight container in the pantry or refrigerator.

haloumi cheese fritters

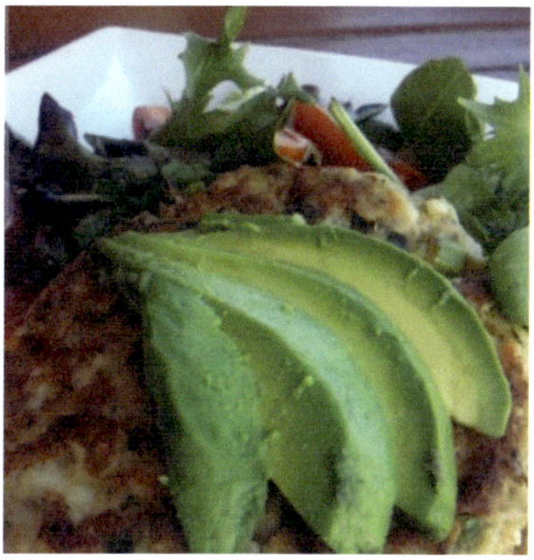

SERVINGS: 4

PREP TIME: 10 mins

COOKING TIME: 15 mins

serving suggestion

Serve hot or cold with food such as avocado, yogurt, poached eggs, rocket.

ingredients

150 g broccoli, roughly chopped

200 g cauliflower, roughly chopped

150 g halloumi cheese, grated

60 g tasty cheese, grated

4 free range eggs, lightly whisked

3 tbsp psyllium seed husks

3 tbsp coconut flour

2 tbsp butter

salt and freshly cracked black pepper to taste

method

Pulse the broccoli and cauliflower in a food processor until finely chopped (or use a cheese grater).

Combine all ingredients in large mixing bowl, then season to taste.

Set aside for 10 minutes to allow the psyllium seed husks to become glutinous and to help bind the mixture together.

Heat some butter in a large frying pan over a medium heat.

Using clean hands, mould the mixture into palm sized fritters before adding to the pan.

Cook the fritters for 3-4 minutes on each side, or until golden.

egg wrap

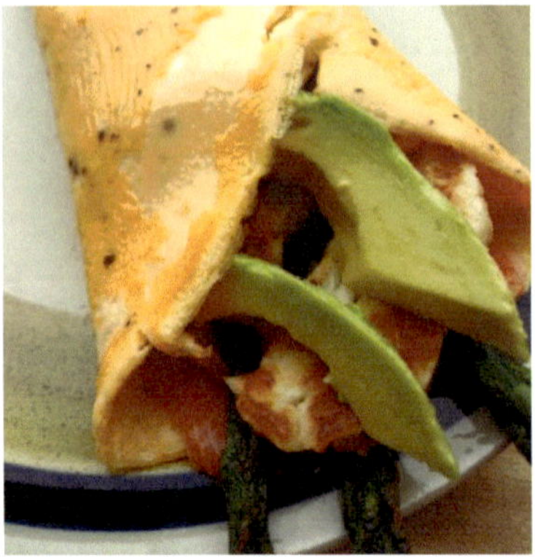

SERVINGS: 1

PREP TIME: 2 mins

COOKING TIME: 5 mins

serving suggestion

Garnish with parsley.

wrap ingredients

2 eggs

1 tbsp water

1 tbsp butter or ghee (for frying)

salt and pepper to taste

filling ingredients

40 g halloumi cheese (sliced)

3 asparagus spears

1 tsp olive oil

¼ avocado, sliced

2 slices of smoked salmon

method

Pan fry the halloumi and asparagus in the olive oil over medium heat for 2 minutes.

Whisk together the egg wrap ingredients, adding salt and pepper to taste.

Pour egg mixture into a large frypan on a low heat and cook until set, flip the egg wrap if needed.

Let egg wrap cool in the pan before flipping onto a serving plate.

To assemble, lay filling in the centre of the egg wrap, leaving space at the bottom to wrap. Fold in one side, then fold the bottom section, and follow with the remaining side.

sardine cakes

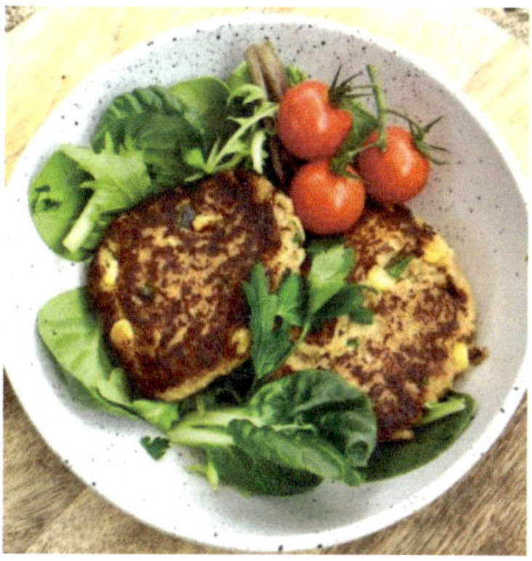

SERVINGS: 6

PREP TIME: 20 mins

COOKING TIME: 10 mins

serving suggestion

Serve with a fresh salad.

ingredients

1 small sweet potato

4 spring onions

¼ cup corn

200 g sardines, drained

1 egg

1 tbsp psyllium husks

salt and pepper

method

Dice the sweet potato and boil until it softens.

Drain oil from canned sardines and add to a bowl; add sliced spring onions, corn, and salt and pepper, mixing all together.

Once sweet potato is softened, drain and mash.

Add mashed sweet potato into the sardine mixture, add the psyllium and egg and mix well. Let sit for 5 minutes.

Shape sardine mixture into palm sized patties.

Fry sardine cakes over medium heat in frypan with a dash of olive oil until cooked through.

mexican beans

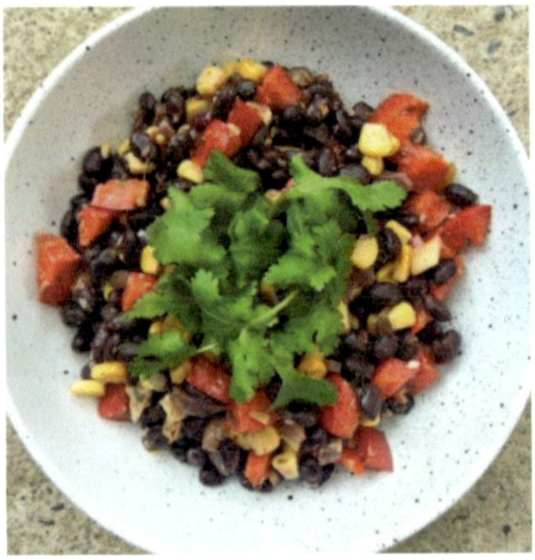

SERVINGS: 4

PREP TIME: 5 mins

COOK TIME: 15 mins

serving suggestion

Add garnish and serve.

ingredients

1 small red onion

1 tbsp olive oil

1 red capsicum, diced

2 cans of black beans, drained and rinsed

1 can of corn kernels

2 tbsp crushed garlic

1 tsp ground cumin seeds

1 tsp ground chili flakes

1 tsp dried coriander leaves

salt to taste

method

Slice red onion and add to a frypan with olive oil, cook until softened. Add the remaining ingredients and stir/simmer for 10 minutes.

garnish

With cayenne pepper and fresh coriander.

sweet potato toasty

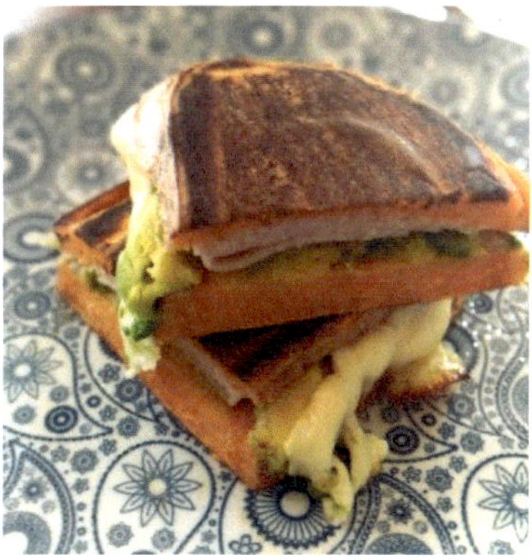

SERVINGS: 1

PREP TIME: 3 mins

COOKING TIME: variable

serving suggestion

Serve with a side of fresh salad.

ingredients

2 slices of sweet potato

¼ avocado

2 slices of ham

2 slices of red onion

2 slices tasty cheese

dash of olive oil

method

Slice 2 portions of sweet potato length ways.

Layer one side with ham, cheese, avocado, and red onion and add the other slice of sweet potato on the layers.

Rub some olive oil into top and bottom sides.

Toast in a sandwich press until cooked through.

DINNER

lamb cutlet one tray bake

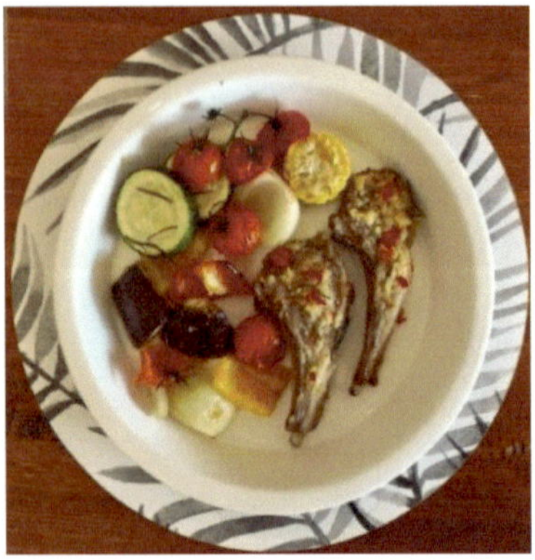

SERVINGS: 3

PREP TIME: 10 mins

COOKING TIME: 25 mins

serving suggestion

Serve with cumin spiced yoghurt dressing. *(recipe next page)*

ingredients

6 lamb cutlets

1 tbsp minced garlic

1 lemon, juice and rind

1 tbsp olive oil

1 red chilli, chopped finely

½ cob corn, chopped in half

½ small eggplant

½ zucchini

½ yellow capsicum

½ red capsicum

¼ brown onion

6 cherry tomatoes

2 sprigs fresh rosemary

salt and pepper to taste

method

Preheat oven to 180°C.

Add garlic, lemon juice and rind, olive oil, chili, salt and pepper to a bowl to make a marinade.

Coat lamb well in marinade.

Slice vegetables into thick slices/chunks and add some olive oil, add seasoning of choice, mixing in a bowl.

Lay marinated lamb into a baking dish, top with vegetables, and cherry tomatoes. Top with remaining marinade.

Sprinkle with fresh rosemary and bake for 25-30 minutes.

cumin spiced yogurt dressing

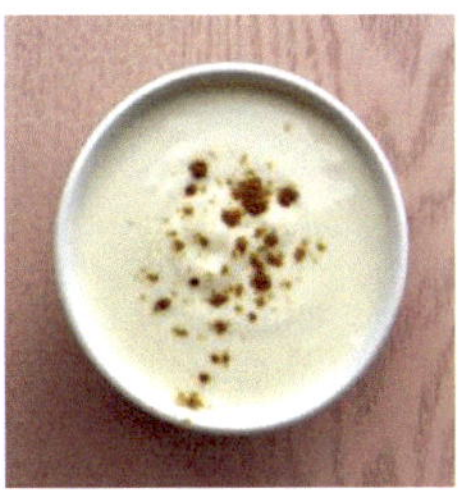

serving suggestion

Serve with lamb cutlet one tray bake.
(recipe previous page)

ingredients

4 tbsp Greek yoghurt

1 tbsp honey

1 tsp ground cumin

method

Stir all ingredients together and serve chilled.

olive and fish one pan bake

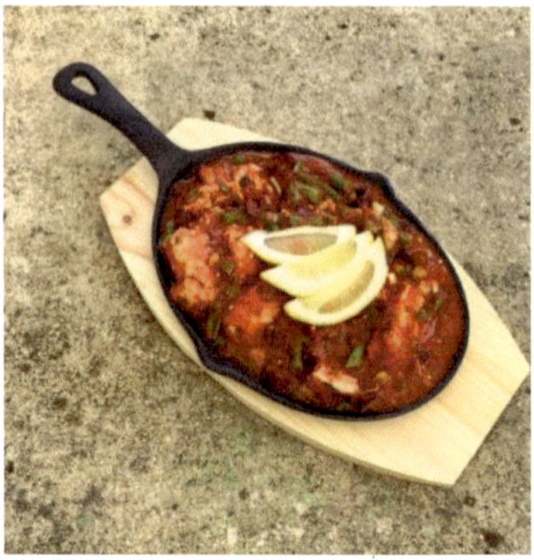

SERVINGS: 4

PREP TIME: 5 mins

COOKING TIME: 20 mins

serving suggestion

Serve with fresh green leaves and lemon wedges.

ingredients

450 ml passata tomato puree sauce

2 cloves crushed garlic

4 finely chopped spring onions

200 g sliced black pitted olives

1 cup chopped green beans

1 lemon, ground zest & juice

60 ml olive oil

3 tbsp fresh chopped parsley

500 g white fish e.g. Gummy Shark

1 tsp salt

1 tsp pepper

method

Preheat oven 170 degrees C.

Mix all ingredients together in the baking dish.

Bake for 20-25 minutes.

pumpkin soup

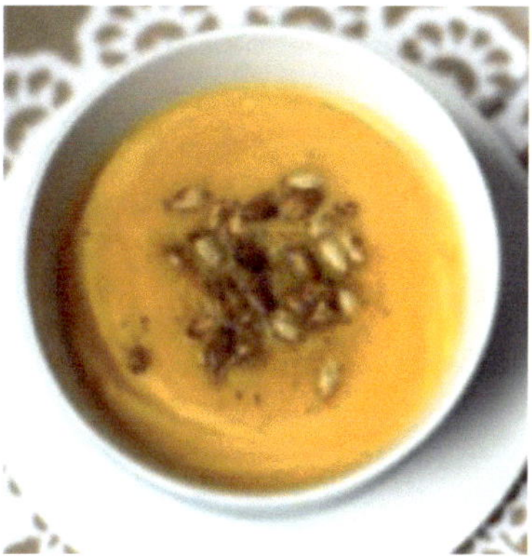

SERVINGS: 6

PREP TIME: 10 mins

COOKING TIME: 40 mins

serving suggestion

Make the most of your pumpkin by roasting the seeds and using as a garnish with sour cream.

ingredients

1 kg pumpkin, roughly chopped

1 carrot, roughly chopped

1 onion, roughly chopped

2 cloves garlic, minced

1 tbsp olive oil

dried chilli flakes (optional)

sea salt and freshly cracked black pepper

1L chicken or vegetable stock

method

Preheat the oven to 180°C.

Place the pumpkin, carrot, onion and garlic in a large baking dish and drizzle with olive oil.

Season to taste, then bake in the oven for 25-30 minutes, or until the pumpkin is soft and

starting to caramelise.

Transfer the roasted vegetables to a large stock pot, add the stock, then blend with a stick blender until smooth.

Heat the soup over a medium heat and serve warm.

Garnish each bowl with sour cream, roasted pumpkin seeds and freshly cracked black pepper.

stuffed eggplant boats

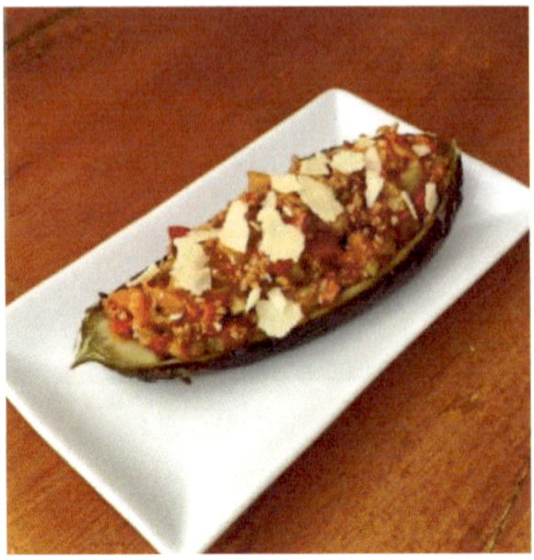

SERVINGS: 4

PREP TIME: 15 mins

COOKING TIME: 2 hours

serving suggestion

Serve sprinkled with basil leaves.

ingredients

eggplant boats

2 (500 g each) eggplants

2 tbsp extra virgin olive oil

⅔ cup shredded fresh basil leaves

1 cup shaved parmesan

bolognese sauce

2 tbsp extra virgin olive oil

1 tbsp chopped fresh oregano

1 tbsp chopped fresh parsley

1 tbsp chopped fresh basil

1 medium brown onion, finely chopped

2 garlic cloves, crushed

2 large carrots, finely chopped

1 large red capsicum, finely chopped

4 celery stalks, finely chopped

500 g beef mince

1 x 400 g can diced tomatoes

2 tbsp tomato paste

2 tsp salt

method

prepare eggplant

Preheat oven to 180°C fan forced and line a baking tray with baking paper.

Pierce eggplant several times with a fork. Cover all over with oil.

Place on prepared tray. Bake for 40 minutes or until tender. Cool slightly.

Cut eggplants in half lengthways.

Using a spoon, scoop flesh from the eggplant halves, leaving a 1cm border.

Finely chop flesh.

prepare bolognese sauce

Heat oil in a large saucepan over medium heat.

Add onion, garlic, carrot, capsicum and celery, mixed herbs.

Cook, stirring, for 5 minutes or until onion has softened.

Add mince. Cook, stirring with a wooden spoon to break up mince, for 5 minutes or until browned.

Add tomatoes, salt and tomato paste. Bring to the boil. Reduce heat to low.

Simmer, covered, for 30 minutes.

Remove cover. Simmer for 20 to 25 minutes or until thickened.

assemble

Combinc Bolognese, shredded basil and chopped eggplant in a medium bowl.

Place eggplant halves on baking tray.

Spoon Bolognese mixture into eggplant.

Sprinkle with parmesan.

Bake for 20 minutes or until heated through.

Nutrition for life!

Meal Planner – 1 week – Mediterranean Diet

		MONDAY	TUESDAY	WEDNESDAY	THURSDAY	FRIDAY	SATURDAY	SUNDAY
Breakfast	Food:	Acai Smoothie Bowl	Fruit and Yogurt	Haloumi Fritters	Poached egg on sourdough	Granola and Yogurt	Berry smoothie	Veggie omelette
Lunch	Food:	Egg wrap with smoked salmon	Sweet potato toastie	Minestrone soup	Sardine cakes with salad	Spicy Mexican beans	Kaleslaw with hummus	Greek salad with tuna
Dinner	Food:	Mediterranean lamb cutlet bake	Spinach and feta quiche	Chicken cacciatore	Portobello mushroom pizzas	One pan olive and fish bake	Eggplant bolognaise boats	Pumpkin soup

LIST OF ILLUSTRATIONS, PHOTOGRAPHS, TABLES

ACCESS TO INTERVIEWS AND FURTHER INFORMATION

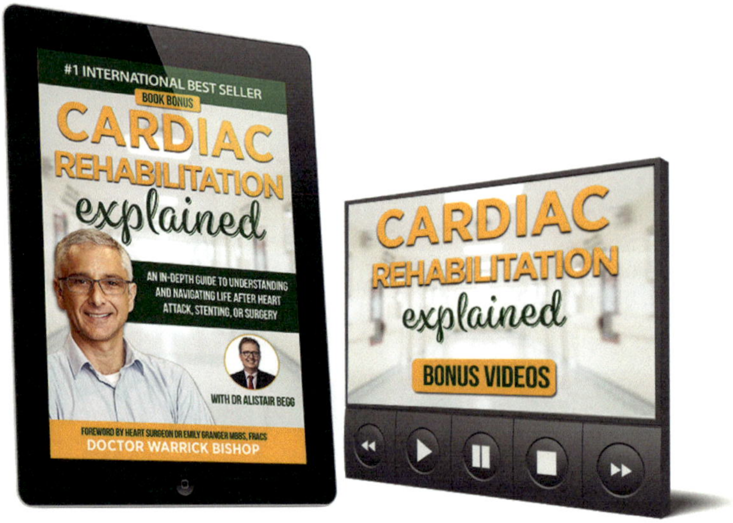

interviews

- Alistair Begg, *cardiologist, rehabilitation specialist*
- Angela Hartley, *cardiac rehabilitation services provider*
- Ashutosh Hardikar, *cardiothoracic surgeon*
- Brian, patient and surfer
- Darren Lehmann, *cricketer*
- Greg Page, *entertainer*
- Ralf Ilchef, *liaison psychiatrist*
- Robert Zecchin, *cardiac rehabilitation clinician-researcher*
- *PDF Checklists*

bonus videos

- Drugs used in cardiology
- Do I need to take medications forever
- If I've had a problem what about my family

SCAN ME

other books by dr warrick bishop

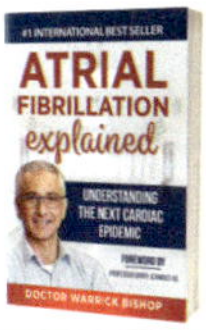

Atrial Fibrillation Explained: *a comprehensive guide that provides an easy-to-understand overview of atrial fibrillation, covering its causes, symptoms, and treatment options.*

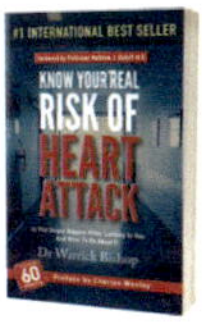

Know Your Real Risk of Heart Attack: *Texplains the various risk factors that contribute to heart disease and provides practical advice on how to reduce your risk, making it an excellent resource for anyone looking to take control of their heart health.*

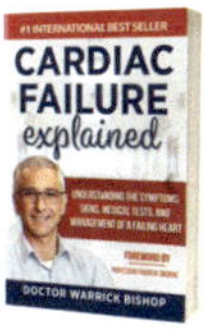

Cardiac Failure Explained*: a complete guide to understanding and managing heart failure, covering everything from the causes and symptoms of heart failure to the latest treatment options available.*

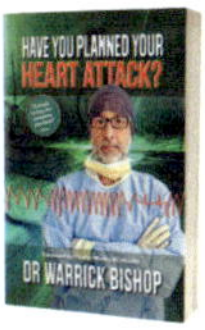

Have You Planned Your Heart Attack?: *offers a balanced and referenced discussion of coronary risk assessment using modern technology, specifically CT scans to evaluate the health of coronary arteries*

Find out more at: *https://drwarrickbishop.com/page/books*

courses & memberships:

Weight Loss Course: *https://healthyheartnetwork.com/page/weightloss*

Atrial Fibrillation Kit: *https://drwarrickbishop.com/page/atrial-fibrillation-explained-premium-kit*

Healthy Heart Network Membership: *https://healthyheartnetwork.com*

other resources:

Heart Attacks are Preventable Webinar: *https://healthyheartnetwork.com*

How Healthy is Your Heart, Really? *https://virtualheartcheck.com.au*

Download our free Mobile App: *https://healthyheartnetwork.com/page/mobile*

GLOSSARY

A

aldosterone
a mineralocorticoid produced in the renin-angiotensin-aldosterone system (RAAS) that acts at the distal tubule, retaining sodium and therefore water, thus keeping up the fluid level

aldosterone blocker/antagonist
blocks the renin-angiotensin-aldosterone system (RAAS), releasing sodium and water, which then passes from the body as urine; most used drugs are spironolactone and eplerenone

angiogram
contrast (dye) injected into a patient that outlines the coronary arteries in exquisite detail, giving information about the location, the quality and nature of the plaque, the degree of stenosis and the size of the vessel affected. There are two types of coronary angiogram:

> **CT coronary angiogram** or a CCTA, a coronary computed tomography angiogram, which is non-invasive, and
>
> **'invasive' angiogram** as it requires a small tube to be passed from an artery in the arm or leg to the heart to inject dye directly into the arteries

angiotensin II (AT2)
works on the angiotensin II receptor and causes vasoconstriction – keeps up the blood pressure; dilates the kidney's efferent arteriole and so reduces filtration. The resultant fluid overload places a strain on the heart that could be detrimental to a heart in cardiac failure

angiotensin II (AT2) receptor
drives much of the action within the renin-angiotensin-aldosterone system (RAAS), including the production of aldosterone

angiotensin II (AT2) receptor blocker (ARB)
acts directly on the AT2 receptor in the renin-angiotensin-aldosterone system (RAAS), releasing sodium and water, which then passes from the body as urine; lowers blood pressure, constricts efferent arteriole, lessens aldosterone production. Commonly used drugs are candesartan, telmisartan and valsartan. Should not be given with ACE inhibitors, although they are interchangeable

angiotensin-converting enzyme (ACE)
the enzyme that converts angiotensin I (AT1) to angiotensin II (AT2)

angiotensin-converting enzyme (ACE) inhibitor
blocks the renin-angiotensin-aldosterone system (RAAS) – prevents the conversion of AT1 to AT2 – releasing sodium and water, which then passes from the body as urine. Used for patients whose hearts are not pumping well – hearts with reduced ejection fraction (HFrEF). Current commonly used drugs include enalapril, perindopril and ramipril. Should not be given with ARBs, although they are interchangeable

anticoagulant
a blood thinner that slows down the formation of a clot and so helps reduce the risk of a clot forming; common agents are warfarin, heparin and non-vitamin K oral anticoagulants

antiplatelet
blood thinner that prevents blood components – platelets – from clumping together; helps reduce the risk of a clot forming; common agents are aspirin and clopidogrel

atrial fibrillation (AF)
an 'irregularly irregular' heartbeat, characterised by the loss of the coordinated contraction of the top part of the heart, the atrial chambers, or atria. It affects the pumping capacity of the heart. The condition can be managed but not cured. AF distinctions:

> **overt or symptomatic** AF
> the type the patient can feel
>
> **silent or asymptomatic** AF
> the type the patient cannot feel and is discovered as an incidental finding
>
> **paroxysmal** AF
> lasts between 24 and 48 hours but no longer than a week
>
> **persistent** AF
> lasts longer than seven days
>
> **permanent** AF
> is present for longer than a year
>
> **valvular** AF
> if the patient has a narrow mitral valve or artificial heart valve; is associated with a greater risk of a clot forming in the left atrial appendage

arteries
the vessels of the body's circulation system that carry the blood away from the heart

> **aorta**
> the biggest artery of the body, takes the blood from the left ventricle as the blood begins its journey around the body. Coming from the aorta as it leaves the heart are
>
> > the **right coronary artery** (RCA) which provides blood to the surface of the heart, the area nearest the diaphragm, and
> >
> > the **left main coronary artery** (LM) which divides into
> >
> > > the **left anterior descending artery** (LAD) and provides blood to the anterior surface of the heart, the area nearest the chest wall, and
> > >
> > > the **circumflex artery** which provides blood to the back of the heart, the area nearest the spine
>
> **coronary arteries**
> are the first branches in the body's circulation system and supply oxygenated blood to the heart muscle
>
> **carotid arteries**
> a pair of major blood vessels in the neck that deliver blood to the brain and head
>
> **left internal mammary artery (LIMA)**
> an artery behind the sternum that supplies blood to the chest wall; considered a conduit of choice in coronary artery bypass graft (CABG) surgery. Also known as the internal thoracic artery (ITA)

radial artery
supplies blood to the forearm and the hand; can be used as the conduit in coronary artery bypass graft (CABG) surgery

associations
connected, joined or related to

asymptomatic
producing or showing no symptoms

atrium
a pre-pumping chamber of the heart. There is an atrium on each side of the heart

the **right atrium** moves blood from the body through the right ventricle to the lungs,

the **left atrium** moves blood from the lungs through the left ventricle into the body.

automaticity
an automatic depolarisation system of the cells of the heart

B

beta-blockers
drugs frequently used to control the heart rate. They

dampen the over-drive effect of the sympathetic nervous system which has nerve endings supplying the AV node, reducing the speed of electrical conduction from the atria to the ventricles and thus slowing the heart rate, and

target the high density of beta receptors (specifically beta2 receptors) in the heart;

improve mortality, morbidity and quality of life for people with reduced cardiac function

commonly used drugs are metoprolol, carvedilol, bisoprolol, extended-release metoprolol and nebivolol

bisoprolol
a commonly-use beta-blocker; others include carvedilol, extended-release metoprolol and nebivolol

blood
the bodily fluid that transports oxygen and nutrients to the body and removes carbon dioxide and other waste. Among its components are platelets (which help in clot formation)

blood clot (thrombus)
a soft, thick lump comprising platelets and fibrin to prevent blood loss if a blood vessel is damaged. A clot can also form inside an artery or vein and stop or block the normal flow of blood. This situation can be very dangerous. If it dislodges and travels though the circulatory system, this is called embolization and can cause a major disaster within the body, such as stroke, pulmonary embolism, deep vein thrombosis (DVT), kidney failure or pregnancy complications

blood flow restoration
procedures to restore blood flow to blocked arteries that include the implantation of a stent/s or bypass grafting

C

calcium channel blocker
stops calcium from entering the cells of the heart and the arteries; used for high blood pressure, chest pain and irregular heartbeat; common agents include nifedipine and amlodipine (peripherally-active) and diltiazem and verapamil (centrally-active); agents best avoided in the presence of cardiac failure

candesartan
a commonly used AT2 receptor blocker (ARB); can be used for high blood pressure. Valsartan and telmisartan are other commonly used ARBs

captopril
the first of the angiotensin-converting enzyme (ACE-I) inhibitors, a powerful agent developed in the 1990s for the treatment and management of congestive heart failure in people with decreased LV function, or reduced contraction of the heart. Its use provides improved quality of life, morbidity and mortality. Later, similar drugs include enalapril, perindopril and ramipril

cardiac arrest
occurs when the electrical impulses of the heart malfunction, leaving the heart unable to pump blood to the body. The symptoms are immediate, with the person non-responsive and not breathing. It can happen to anyone at any time. The causes vary. Without immediate action (CPR and defibrillation), only a small percentage of sufferers survive

cardiac failure (CF)
the heart does not pump as well as it should, leading to a complex mix of a sick heart, maladapted responses to impaired circulation and fluid retention that further strains the heart into a downward spiral of deterioration

cardiac failure, acute
when the heart fails, suddenly; a medical emergency

cardiac imaging
any method used to image the muscle, valves and arteries of the heart

> **echocardiography** – assesses dynamic function of muscle and valves
>
> **CT imaging** – assesses the health and structure of the arteries in a non-invasive way
>
> **invasive angiography** – provides the clearest picture of the narrowing of the arteries
>
> **magnetic resonance imaging** (MRI)/ **cardiac magnetic resonance** (CMR) – shows scarring within the heart and inflammation, in exquisite detail
>
> **nuclear medicine** – assesses aspects of cellular function, blood flow and heart function

cardio-pulmonary resuscitation (CPR)
is an emergency lifesaving technique, of hard and fast chest compressions in association with mouth-to-mouth resuscitation, used when someone's breathing or heartbeat has stopped. Even if untrained and uncertain about what to do, it is always better to try something than to do nothing. The difference between doing something and doing nothing could be someone's life

cardiovascular disease (CVD)
general term for conditions affecting the heart or blood vessels; includes coronary heart disease, angina, heart attack, congenital heart disease, stroke and vascular dementia

coronary artery bypass graft (CABG)
a major surgical procedure used to treat coronary artery disease (CAD), in which part of a healthy vein or artery is used to divert blood around narrowed or clogged arteries to improve blood flow to the heart muscle

coronary artery disease (CAD) or **coronary heart disease** (CHD)
the process of atherosclerosis, or plaque build-up, in the artery that leads to a narrowing of the artery and reduced blood flow. If left undetected, this can produce symptoms including angina, shortness of breath, and lead to a heart attack

carvedilol
a commonly-used beta-blocker; others include bisoprolol, extended-release metoprolol and nebivolol

causations
factors/actions that cause the problem

CHADS / CHA2DS2-VA score
indicates the risk of stroke; used in atrial fibrillation management decisions

co-morbidities
other serious conditions suffered concurrently with the primary health problem

D

dapagliflozin
sodium-glucose transport inhibitor (SGLT2 inhibitor); see gliflozin

depression
a common illness worldwide that is characterised by severe and prolonged low mood; is different to usual mood fluctuations and short-lived emotional responses to challenges in everyday life. The affected person can suffer greatly and function poorly. At worst, it can lead to suicide.

diltiazem
a calcium channel blocker that should be avoided in the presence of cardiac failure; also verapamil

disease
a symptom or loss of normal function

distal
situated away from the centre

diuretic
medication to make a patient pass fluid – relieves congestion and reduces strain on the heart

diuretic, loop
medication that works by blocking the concentrating mechanisms within the loop of the renal tubule, the Loop of Henle; the most used drug is furosemide (frusemide)

dual antiplatelet therapy (DAPT)
two drugs, such as aspirin and clopidogrel, which block platelet function, used together as a blood-thinning therapy after stent implantation

E

echocardiogram (echo)
echo, sound, *cardio*, heart, *gram*, picture
a scan of the heart using ultrasound waves to acquire a picture. It gives information about the valves, the chambers of the heart and pressures within the heart

electrocardiogram (ECG)
a trace of the electrical activity through the heart acquired by electrodes. It shows the rhythm of the heart. Features of an ECG can be used to determine the status of the heart muscle.

> **P wave**
> electrical activity in the atria, reflecting actual depolarization or the electrical flow. No P wave with chaotic electrical activity is the diagnostic thumbprint of atrial fibrillation
>
> **QRS complex**
> created by the electrical impulses reflecting the depolarisation of the major muscle of the heart
>
> **T wave**
> the return of normal repolarization to the heart muscle ready for the next beat

empagliflozin
a gliflozin or sodium-glucose transport inhibitor (SGLT2 inhibitor)

enalapril
one of the ACE inhibitor drugs currently used in the treatment and management of congestive heart failure in people with decreased left ventricle function, or reduced contraction of the heart; providing improved quality of life, morbidity and mortality; other similar drugs include perindopril, ramipril and captopril

eplerenone
a common aldosterone antagonist that works on the distal tubule

extracorporeal membrane oxygenation (ECMO)
a machine, very similar to a bypass machine, that takes blood from the patient to transfer oxygen through a membrane outside the body to maintain oxygenation to the person; used for critically unwell patients with a good chance of recovery

F

furosemide (frusemide)
one of the most used loop diuretic drugs

G

gliflozin
the sodium-glucose transport inhibitor (SGLT2 inhibitor) that

> works at the proximal tubule of the kidney, allowing salt and water to be lost through the urine; developed initially to aid diabetics
>
> reduces hospitalizations
>
> improves quality of life especially for diabetic patients with CF, and
>
> improves mortality;

the first drug identified to provide benefit in cardiac failure was empagliflozin, while a 2019 report to the European Society of Cardiology showed that the drug, dapagliflozin, was a beneficial add-on therapy for cardiac failure patients already appropriately treated regardless of whether or not they had diabetes. The SGLTs-1 drugs are now included as routine therapy for patients with reduced ejection fraction cardiac failure

glucagon-like peptide-1 receptor antagonist (GLP-1 RA)
a drug for diabetes that appears to reduce cardiac events; agents include semaglutide, dulaglutide and exenatide

H

HAS-BLED score
indicates risk of bleeding; used in atrial fibrillation management decisions

heart
a large muscle that pumps blood through the body

heart attack
a non-medical expression. It is a layman's term referring to a

myocardial infarction

myo, muscle, *cardio*, heart, *infarction*, death by lack of blood flow

most commonly, but not always, it is caused by the narrowing of the coronary arteries that can kill or requires some form of medical intervention – medication, time in hospital, balloons or stents, or coronary artery bypass grafting. There are two types of heart attack:

NSTEMI – non -ST-Elevation Myocardial Infarction, in which the coronary artery is partially and temporarily blocked

STEMI – ST-Elevation Myocardial Infarction, in which the coronary artery is completely and permanently blocked

The type of heart attack is determined by the results of the ECG. While the NSTEMI is the less serious of the two because less damage is done to the heart, it is still a serious condition that requires immediate diagnosis and treatment

L

Loop of Henle
a region between the proximal and distal tubules of the kidney where concentration of urine may occur; a region where certain diuretic drugs (loop diuretics) work

M

metoprolol
a commonly-used beta-blocker, for heart rate control; others include bisoprolol, carvedilol and nebivolol; available in an extended-release preparation for CF

mineralocorticoid
mineralo, mineral balance; *corticoids*, steroid-based hormones

hormone messengers that influence electrolyte and water balance in the body; the primary mineralocorticoid is aldosterone

mineralocorticoid blocker
can be used as a diuretic. If used in conjunction with a loop diuretic, particular care needs to be exercised around fluid balance and fluid loss, with regular blood testing and clinical assessment essential

myocardium
myo, muscle, *cardium*, being of the heart

the muscle of the heart

N

nebivolol
a commonly-used beta-blocker; others include bisoprolol, carvedilol and extended-release metoprolol

neprilysin inhibitor
helps stop the breakdown of the natriuretic peptides (good guys); cannot be used in conjunction with ACE inhibitors; most commonly used drug, sacubitril

nitrates
relax the blood vessels and reduce the load on the heart; cannot be used with Viagra-type preparations; commonly used agents are based on isosorbide mononitrate

nodes

sinoatrial (SA) node
a cluster of specialised heart cells located in the top of the right atrium and it is where the electrical activity of the heart originates and drives the rhythm of the heart

atrioventricular (AV) node
a cluster of cells in the centre of the heart between the atria and ventricles that allows electrical communication; also acts as a gatekeeper, regulating the electrical impulses as they come from the atria and enter the ventricles

non-vitamin K anticoagulants (NOAC)
relatively new, fast-acting anticoagulants; commonly used agents are apixaban, dabigatran and rivaroxaban

P

palpitations
arrhythmic, or irregular, heartbeats

rapid and irregular

atrial (top of the heart) **ectopic** (out of place) **beats** (heartbeat)
extra beats arising from the top part of the heart

ventricular ectopic beats
extra beats arising from the ventricle

rapid and regular

atrial flutter
similar to atrial fibrillation except that the heart beat is regular and there is a re-entrant circuit occurring in the right atrium

supraventricular tachycardia
supra, above the ventricle, *tachy*, fast, *cardia*, pertaining to the heart
an electrical short circuit in the atria that keeps firing on itself

ventricular tachycardia
a high-risk rhythm in the main pumping chamber of the heart

ventricular fibrillation
a cause of sudden cardiac death

perindopril
one of the ACE inhibitor drugs currently used in the treatment and management of congestive heart failure in people with decreased left ventricle function, or reduced contraction of the heart; providing improved quality of life, morbidity and mortality; other similar drugs include, enalapril, ramipril and captopril

prognostic (prognosis)
improving the long-term outcome for the patient

proximal
situated near the centre

R

ramipril
one of the ACE inhibitor drugs currently used in the treatment and management of congestive heart failure in people with decreased LV function, or reduced contraction of the heart; providing improved quality of life, morbidity and mortality; other similar drugs include enalapril, perindopril and captopril

renin-angiotensin-aldosterone system (RAAS)
the chemical messenger system that regulates blood pressure through the kidneys; produces aldosterone (keeps sodium in the kidneys – increases fluid volume in the body)

renin-angiotensin-aldosterone system (RAAS) **blocker**
releases sodium and water, which pass out of the body as urine. Therapies include angiotensin-converting enzyme (ACE) inhibitors, angiotensin II (AT2) receptor blockers, aldosterone blockers

rhythm

sinus (normal)
the healthy heart rhythm, which is controlled by the sinoatrial, or sinus, node, beating in asynchronistic and smooth manner

arrhythmia
when the synchronicity of the heartbeat breaks down

S

sodium-glucose transport inhibitor (SGLT2)
see gliflozin

spironolactone
a common aldosterone antagonist that works on the distal tubule in the kidney

stenosis
narrowing

stenting
a mechanical intervention for coronary artery disease in which an intravascular device (balloon) within a wire scaffold is inserted percutaneously (through the skin) and guided to the site of the narrowing. When the balloon is inflated, the artery is opened. When the balloon is removed, the wire scaffold remains to keep it open. The scaffold is called a stent

stress test
a test of heart function. It involves exercising the patient or giving the patient medication to replicate exercise, to try to reproduce the symptom under investigation or unmask areas where there is a lack of blood flow to the heart

stroke
a disruption of the blood supply to the brain leading to permanent loss of function

> **haemorrhagic**
> when a blood vessel ruptures and bleeds into the brain
>
> **ischemic**
> when a clot (also called thrombus) blocks an artery, leading to a lack of blood flow. Such clots often form in the large blood vessels in the neck, the carotid arteries, or in the heart because of atrial fibrillation

sublingual glyceryl trinitrate (GTN)
a spray under the tongue, to be used when a person experiences chest pain (angina); it is given with some caution; not to be used with Viagra

symptomatic improvement
improving how the patient feels

T

telmisartan
a commonly used AT2 receptor blocker (ARB); can be used for blood pressure. Candesartan and valsartan are other commonly used ARBs

troponin
a protein found in the heart that is leaked into the blood when the heart is damaged or stressed. A blood test to measure troponin is used as a predictor when a person presents with chest pain to assess the likelihood of the heart being involved

thiazides
a mainstay of blood pressure therapy, they

> block the sodium (salt) retaining function of the distal convoluted tubule in the kidney (the resulting salt and water loss reduces blood volume and so lowers blood pressure) and
>
> lower blood pressure by dilating (relaxing or widening) the blood vessels

V

valsartan
a commonly used AT2 receptor blocker (ARB); can be used for high blood pressure. Candesartan and telmisartan are other commonly used ARBs

valves
keep blood flowing through the heart in the right direction

(in order of blood flow)

> **tricuspid**
> a one-way valve between the right atrium and the right ventricle
>
> **pulmonary**
> a one-way valve between the right ventricle and the pulmonary circulation, which takes the blood to the lungs
>
> **mitral**
> a one-way valve between the left atrium and the left ventricle
>
> **aortic**
> a one-way valve between the left ventricle and the aorta, which is the main artery leading from the heart into the body

valve repair/replacement
the mitral valve and the aortic valve, both on the left side of the heart, can become too tight (stenosis) or leak (regurgitation or incompetence)

> **mitral valve**
> can be repaired (preferred) or replaced using metallic or biological tissue
>
> **aortic valve**
> can be replaced either by open-heart surgery or for a tight aortic valve, by minimally invasive technology called transcutaneous aortic valve implantation (TAVI)

veins
low pressure blood vessels that mostly carry deoxygenated blood towards the heart. The ones that most concern us are:

> **IVC, inferior vena cava**
> is one of two major veins that drains into the right atrium; it collects blood flowing below the heart
>
> **jugular vein**
> carries blood from the brain, face and neck, and connects with the SVC to take the blood to the right atrium; a 'dipstick' for fluid pressure in the right atrium (the waveform of the jugular pulse is often visible in patients with a sick heart when sitting upright)
>
> **pulmonary veins**
> are the exception, and the four pulmonary veins transfer oxygenated blood from the lungs to the left atrium of the heart
>
> **saphenous vein** (the great saphenous vein, GSV)
> is the longest vein in the body; part of the vein, taken from the calf or thigh, is a commonly used medium in coronary artery bypass graft (CABG) surgery, with a 40-50 per cent failure rate after 10 years

SVC, superior vena cava
is one of two major veins that drains into the right atrium; it collects blood flowing above the heart

ventricle
the main compression (pumping) chamber of the heart that pushes the blood through the body. There is a right and the left ventricle

right ventricle
pumps the oxygen-poor blood into the lungs

left ventricle (the main pumping chamber of the heart)
pumps oxygen-rich blood into the body

verapamil
a calcium channel blocker that should be avoided in the presence of cardiac failure; also diltiazem

viable heart muscle
heart muscle that is not receiving enough blood but is still alive; also known as hibernating myocardium

INDEX

D

ACKNOWLEDGEMENTS AND THANKS

A book such as this doesn't 'just happen'. Obviously, it needs time. More importantly, though, it needs a variety of people with different skills and experiences to mine to flesh out what starts as a possibility, an idea.

Cardiac Rehabilitation Explained requires three additions to the list of people who support me in bringing a book such as this into existence.

Firstly, my collaborator and co-author, colleague and friend, **Alistair Begg,** a cardiologist with a special interest in rehabilitation who initially headed me in this direction and then provided valuable assistance and insight into the material of the book itself.

Secondly, a group of heart event sufferers – **Ron, Brian, Darren Lehmann,** and **Greg Page** – and rehabilitation specialists – **Ashutosh Hardikar, Robert Zecchin, Angela Hartley,** and **Ralf Ilchef** – who participated in Healthy Heart Network interviews with me and graciously and generously allowed their personal and professional experiences to be featured throughout these pages. This personal insight adds a new dimension to this, my fourth book.

Thirdly, **Carolyn Astley,** president of the Australian Cardiovascular Health and Rehabilitation Services, and several of her ACRA associates, who provided detailed, beneficial, and valued comment on an early draft of the book.

I also acknowledge my colleagues whom I hold in the highest regard and who were generous in offering professional review and collegial encouragement. Special mention is made of cardiothoracic and heart and lung transplant surgeon **Emily Granger**, of Sydney, New South Wales, for bringing her vast practical and academic experience to the foreword to this book, and world-renown lipid authority and friend **Karam Kostner**, of Brisbane, Queensland.

I'm grateful to my **patients** who have contributed to my collective experience upon which I was able to base this book and to the eagle-eyed masters of detail **David Thomas** and **John Harbinson** who provided candid, invaluable man-in-the-street-comments.

And then there are the highly skilled technical professionals who created the book: designer and artist **Cathy McAuliffe**, master of the computer **Beverly Waldie,** marketer **John North** and his team, and my writing partner **Penny Edman**, each of whom brings talent, commitment, and enthusiasm to the work.

To these close associates, to Chelle and my supportive family, and to everyone else involved in the production of *Cardiac Rehabilitation Explained*, I am deeply grateful.

Warrick Bishop, Hobart, Australia
December 2022

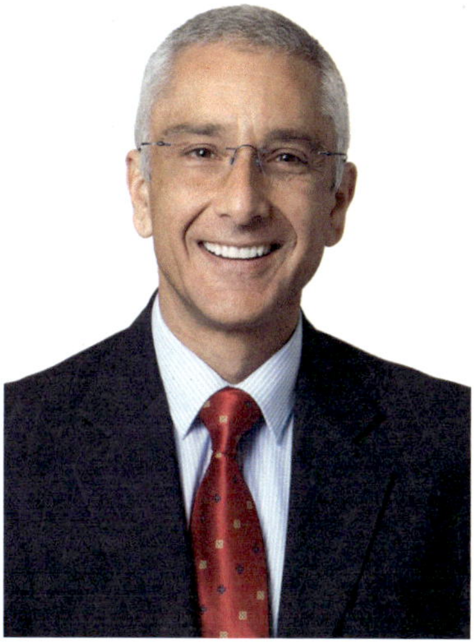

author – **WARRICK BISHOP** is a practising cardiologist with a passion for helping people live as well as possible for as long as possible. He has a special interest in preventing heart attack by using cardiac CT imaging, managing cholesterol, and giving attention to diet. He also supports patients through education as he believes that the best-educated patients receive the best health care.

Warrick graduated from the University of Tasmania, School of Medicine, in 1988. He worked in the Northern Territory before undertaking his specialist training in Adelaide, South Australia. He completed his advanced training in cardiology in Hobart, Tasmania, becoming a fellow of the Royal Australian College of Physicians in 1997. He has worked predominantly in private practice.

In 2009, Warrick undertook training in CT cardiac coronary angiography, becoming the first cardiologist in Tasmania with this specialist recognition. This area of imaging fits well with his interest in preventative cardiology and was the focus of his first book, *Have You Planned Your Heart Attack?* (2016). He is a member of the Society of Cardiovascular Computed Tomography, Australian and New Zealand International Regional Committee (SCCT ANZ IRC).

Warrick is also a member of the Australian Atherosclerosis Society and a participant on the panel of 'interested parties' developing a model of care and a national registry for familial hypercholesterolemia. He has also developed a particular interest in diabetic-related risk of coronary artery disease, specifically allied to eating guidelines and lipid profiles.

Warrick is an accredited examiner for the Royal Australian College of Physicians and is regularly involved with teaching medical students and junior doctors. He has worked on projects, in an affiliate capacity, with Hobart's globally recognised Menzies Institute for Medical Research and has been recognised by the Medical School of the University of Tasmania with academic status.

As a member of the Clinical Issues Committee of the Australian Heart Foundation which provides input into issues of significance for the management of heart patients, Warrick contributed to the Australian Heart Foundation's 2021 position paper on Coronary Artery Calcium.

Warrick enjoys a strong social media profile and in February 2020 he presented a TEDx talk, *Lessons from a Heart Attack*, at Docklands, Victoria, Australia, and then another soon after, *How Medicine, Money and Mindset are Costing Lives*, before a live audience at the University of Mississippi, Jackson, Mississippi, USA.

In addition to authoring numerous articles and the books, *Have You Planned Your Heart Attack?* (published in the USA as *Know Your Real Risk of Heart Attack*), *Atrial Fibrillation Explained, Cardiac Failure Explained*, and now *Cardiac Rehabilitation Explained*, he founded the Healthy Heart Network in 2018.

This book is his first collaborative venture, with fellow cardiologist Dr Alistair Begg, of Adelaide, South Australia.

All of Warrick's public endeavours are aimed at helping people live as well as possible for as long as possible by education and support.

A keen surfer, he enjoys travel and music and playing the guitar with his children.

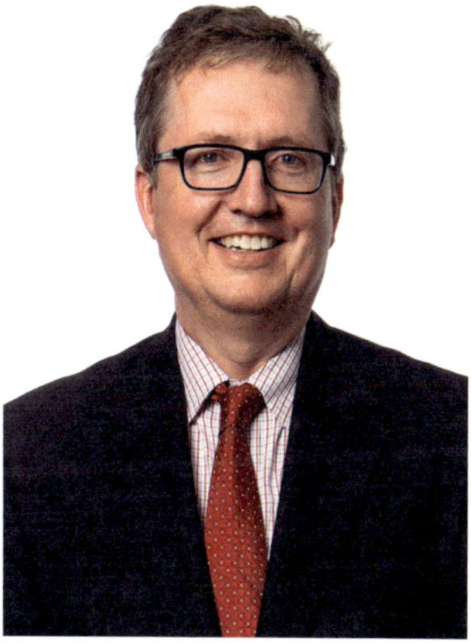

author – **ALISTAIR BEGG** is a skilled cardiologist with expertise in cardiac imaging including exercise stress echocardiography, CT coronary angiography, coronary intervention and general cardiology. Alistair joined SA Heart, a South Australian privately owned and operated specialist cardiology group, in 2007 and regularly consults at the group's Ashford Clinic.

Alistair graduated from Medicine at the University of Adelaide, South Australia, in 1989, and trained in cardiology at Flinders Medical Centre, a public teaching hospital and research centre in Adelaide. During his post-fellowship in Sydney, Alistair specialised in cardiac imaging. In 1996, he was awarded his Fellowship to the Royal Australasian College of Physicians. Alistair obtained his Diploma of Diagnostic Ultrasound in 1997 and, in 2006, he was awarded his Fellowship of the Cardiac Society of Australia and New Zealand. Two years later, he completed level 2 training for CT coronary angiography and enjoys working together with radiology to co-report these tests.

Alistair also has many years of private practice experience in Sydney and Adelaide. His focus is on exercise testing and cardiac imaging. He is particularly interested in patients with chest pain, heart failure, and significant risk factors, and he also places significance on the benefits of diet and exercise in preventing cardiac illness.

He is actively involved in cardiac rehabilitation.

As a schoolboy, an unfortunate tragedy involving a fellow student instilled in Alistair an awareness of the importance of cardiology. Today, he thrives on the ability to detect and treat cardiac conditions. He enjoys being actively involved in research studies with the SA Heart team as this work assists him in keeping abreast of evolving treatments and techniques.

From a young age, Alistair has drawn on his love of sport. Numerous patients are, or have been, elite athletes. He enjoys the challenge of keeping them safe and competitive, from their prime into older age.

When he is not seeing patients, Alistair enjoys watching his son compete in athletics, cycling, and golf, which he would often play from dawn to dusk as a medical student.

writer – **PENELOPE EDMAN** is a freelance writer, editor, high performance coach and photographer based in Hobart, Tasmania, Australia. After beginning her print journalism career in Bundaberg, Queensland, in the late 1970s, she moved to Hobart in 1991. She is an Australasian award-winning journalist and editor, and her articles and photographs have been published throughout Australia and internationally.

She authored four non-fiction books before assisting Dr Bishop with *Have You Planned Your Heart Attack?*, *Atrial Fibrillation Explained*, *Cardiac Failure Explained* and now, also in association with Dr Begg, *Cardiac Rehabilitation Explained*.

As a result of being involved with this book, she had a scan, has taken up walking and is developing improved eating habits.

Made in United States
Troutdale, OR
11/11/2026

57125318R00195